44 0567259 9

Etnical Issues in Advanced

KT-150-890

Commissioning editor: Mary Seager
Desk editor: Deena Burgess
Development editor: Caroline Savage
Production controller: Anthony Read
Cover designer: Fred Rose

Ethical Issues in Advanced Nursing Practice

Edited by
Karen Bartter, MA (Medical Ethics) RN, RM, ADM, Cert Ed.
Senior Lecturer – Midwifery, University of Wolverhampton, UK

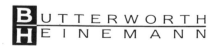

OXFORD   AUCKLAND   BOSTON   JOHANNESBURG   MELBOURNE   NEW DELHI

Butterworth-Heinemann
Linacre House, Jordan Hill, Oxford OX2 8DP
225 Wildwood Avenue, Woburn, MA 01801-2041
A division of Reed Educational and Professional Publishing Ltd

 A member of the Reed Elsevier plc group

First published 2001

British Library Cataloguing in Publication Data
Ethical issues in advanced nursing practice
  1. Nursing ethics
  I. Bartter, Karen
  174.2

ISBN 0 7506 4955 0

For information on all Butterworth-Heinemann nursing
publications visit our website at www.bh.com/nursing

Composition by Genesis Typesetting, Rochester, Kent
Printed and bound in Great Britain by MPG Books Ltd, Bodmin, Cornwall

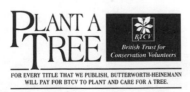

PLANT A TREE
British Trust for Conservation Volunteers

FOR EVERY TITLE THAT WE PUBLISH, BUTTERWORTH-HEINEMANN
WILL PAY FOR BTCV TO PLANT AND CARE FOR A TREE.

Contents

Contributors

Mary Akufo-Tetteh, MSc ACNP, Dip ChN (PN), SRN
Advanced Clinical Nurse Practitioner

Mary works part time in a general practice, she acts as a mentor for the practice nurses within her health authority, and is a Reiki practitioner.

Karen Bartter, MA (Medical Ethics) RN, RM, ADM, Cert Ed
Senior Lecturer – Midwifery, University of Wolverhampton, UK

Karen teaches on a variety of courses from level one to level four, mainly in the topic areas of applied ethics in nursing and midwifery, in both pre- and post-registration courses. As well as teaching applied ethics to nurses on Masters programmes, Karen is also a research supervisor for BSc and Masters level studies. Whilst Karen's present job does not permit a clinical caseload, she does spend some time working with students in the clinical field.

Pamela Campbell, MSc (Advanced Clinical Nursing), PGCE, RHV, RM, RGN, FPCert
Senior Lecturer (Community Nursing), Staffordshire University, UK

Pam worked as an advanced nurse practitioner in a busy general practice surgery before entering the university, where she now teaches on mainly post-registration courses. She is committed to improving the educational opportunities for practice nurses.

June Connolly, MSc ANP, RGN, NP, Dip HE
Advanced Nurse Practitioner in Primary Care

June works as an advanced nurse practitioner in a general medical practice. In addition to running general consultation surgeries, she runs a weekly family planning clinic, with her GP, which is open to the general public. The practice has a cyber café for young people in the local town, and many teenagers attend the practice for contraceptive advice and services.

Alastair Gray, MSc (Advanced Clinical Nursing Practice), BSc (Hons),
RN, DPSN, RNT, ENB199 (Accident and Emergency)
Senior Lecturer (A&E Nursing), University of Wolverhampton, UK

Alastair is the ENB 199 teacher for the A&E departments in the Black Country of the West Midlands. He is committed to advancing nursing practice, and works regularly within a major A&E department in the West Midlands. He is currently developing a lecturer practitioner role.

Karen Harley, MSc ANP, BA(Hons), RGN, RM
Advanced Nurse Practitioner working in General Practice

Karen is currently working as an advanced nurse practitioner in Coventry. She has a particular interest in women's health issues, and is an instructing nurse for family planning students.

Maria Kidd, MSc ANP, RGN, RM, RHV
Health Visitor

Maria carries a health visitor caseload, and holds two nurse practitioner sessions a week within the general practitioner's surgery.

Kate Stuart, MSc ANP, BSc (Hons), RGN
Advanced Nurse Practitioner

Kate works as an advanced nurse practitioner in the Accident and Emergency department at New Cross Hospital, Wolverhampton. Her work includes all aspects of the advanced nurse practitioner role, but she is specifically concerned with clinical practice and educational staff development.

Preface

Advanced nurse practitioners face new and exciting challenges as they push forward the traditional boundaries of nursing, and readily find themselves practising in areas that have traditionally been viewed as part of the doctor's domain.

As such they increasingly have to address challenging ethical issues as the lead professional, and make ethical decisions that may have far-reaching consequences and possibly impact on personal, clinical, legal and professional arenas.

This book seeks to address some of the practical and theoretical dilemmas in advanced nursing practice. It offers the reader a considered background of information for each focus area, and illustrates main points with reflections and application to specific practice issues.

Contributors to the text are primarily advanced nurse practitioners, who studied ethics during their recent MSc Advanced Nurse Practitioner Course and are currently in practice. Their contributions cover a wide range of practice-focused areas, from termination of pregnancy to advance directives, providing relevant and contemporaneous insight and information to advance these debates.

This book will be of value to all qualified and prospective advanced nurse practitioners, including those currently undertaking or facilitating study on an advanced nurse practitioner course, as well as any nurses seeking to advance their practice within an applied ethical contextual framework.

Karen Bartter

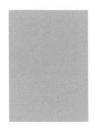

Acknowledgements

In the production of any book there are many people who should be remembered and thanked, and I am sure that each of us involved in this work is grateful to all who have assisted us.

I personally wish to express my thanks to the contributors of this work, for without their hard efforts the book would not exist. I would also like to extend my, and I am sure their, thanks to all the families and friends who have supported, encouraged and generally lived with us through the hours of putting the words on paper.

In addition, my thanks go to Mary Seager and Carrie Savage at Butterworth-Heinemann for invaluable support, guidance and help during this endeavour.

Finally, I would like to dedicate this book to all nurses who strive to advance practice for the benefit of people everywhere; and to my mother, who first inspired me to become a nurse.

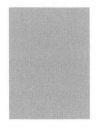

Introduction

To me, ethics is fundamental to life. It is fundamental to all human interactions, and for the advanced nurse practitioner, at the forefront of nursing practice, it is especially important.

Advanced nurse practitioners are the new type of nurses who forge forward, with experience, knowledge and a deeper level of understanding, to cross the traditional boundaries of previous nurse/doctor professional role demarcations. They move forward into largely uncharted waters, with the limited numbers who have gone before them to guide their way and act as knowledgeable and practical supporters. The advanced nurse practitioners of today and tomorrow also have the heavy responsibility of setting the blueprints and standards of advanced practice in their field for the nurses who follow them. They will be and are being judged by others, both professional and lay, for their ability to perform in what has not yet been a unanimously determined role – an arduous task by anyone's standards. Against this demanding backdrop, advanced nurse practitioners serve a more enlightened and autonomous public, who rightly demand excellent standards of care and services from compassionate and intuitive professionals who promote choice and autonomy for their clients.

There is no single font of all wisdom to serve advanced nurse practitioners and others nurses working in advanced practice, and nor indeed could there be. Inspiration, insight and knowledge can and should be gained from a variety of sources. However, we hope that this book, with its collection of chapters on topical themes, will aid all nurses seeking to advance practice.

The main contributors and their peers inspired the book by the work they submitted for assessment during their MSc Advanced Clinical

Nursing Practitioner Course. It occurred to me, as a module leader for one module on that course, that the work submitted by the attending professionals was easily comparable to that already in print. In addition, individuals offered perception and insight into sensitive and current issues affecting their practice and their client groups in today's complex world. Following successful completion of their course, I approached some of those individuals to contribute to this book.

My initial concept was to have only practising advanced nurse practitioners contributing to the chapters; however, there is one small piece by me included in the book. I am not able to speak with the practical authority of a practising advanced nurse practitioner, as my field is as a facilitator of applied ethics in advanced nursing and midwifery education and practice. In Chapter 1, Ethics and Advanced Nursing Practice, I explore the broad issues and expectations of advanced practice, with the conceptual application of principle to practice.

In Chapter 2, June Connolly looks at the legal and ethical implications for the advanced nurse practitioner in relation to contraception and under-16s. She explores the present legal position, considers ethical implications for the advanced nurse practitioner, and gives practitioners guidance in this delicate area. As June says, her work serves to demonstrate 'how law and moral philosophy may intersect and interact with medicine and the future role of the advanced nurse practitioner in general practice'.

Karen Harley believes 'the autonomous role of the advanced nurse practitioner seeking to empower clients through an holistic nursing service will assist in the provision of high quality sexual health care'. Chapter 3 looks at the abortion issue and advanced nursing practice. Here, Karen gives insight to the current legal position and explores related ethical concepts such as the client's individual freedom, autonomy and empowerment, and the advanced nurse practitioner as the client's advocate. She identifies that the advanced practitioner performs activities previously considered as part of the medical domain, but focuses on these with a holistic, caring approach rather than simulating the solely curative medical model.

Continuing in this topic area, in Chapter 4 Pamela Campbell moves her debate into the specific and highly emotive area of termination of pregnancy for fetal abnormality. As Pamela identifies, almost inevitably the advanced nurse practitioner working in primary care will encounter a woman whose fetus is found to be abnormal. Pamela's chapter focuses on ethical considerations and parental support in this situation, and as she states, 'by raising awareness of the issues the advanced nurse practitioner may be better prepared to aid women with their acute and distressing decision making process'.

Maria Kidd's work focuses on the ethical considerations of childhood immunizations and advanced practice. Maria identifies that advanced practitioners must think and function at a more in-depth level. In Chapter 5, she discusses current considerations and offers advanced practitioners working in health visiting practical guidance to assist them in their work in this specific area. As she identifies, there remains a dilemma for practitioners who are 'endeavouring to maintain the autonomy of the individual whilst also considering the greater good of the community'.

In Chapter 6, Kate Stuart focuses on informed consent and advanced practice. Kate considers the legal and ethical position of consent, looking at ethical theories and principles and how all these factors apply in practice. The thorny issue of consent in emergency A&E situations is also considered, and here Kate uses case scenarios to illustrate and explore complex ethical issues.

The practice location of A&E is continued in Chapter 7, where Alastair Gray focuses on the advanced nurse practitioner and empowerment in witnessed resuscitation of relatives. Ethical principles and moral applications are explored in this highly emotive topic area, with associated practical and human considerations being logically and thoughtfully discussed. Guidance is also given to advanced practitioners and A&E staff to assist in the exploration of this topic area.

Chapter 8 is by Mary Akufo-Tetteh, who explores advance directives and considerations for advanced nurse practitioners. Mary starts by giving an overview of the history of advance directives, progressing to how they are used, and their current legal position. Ethical and practical considerations are then explored, and Mary uses two case scenarios to illustrate the practical application of advance directives and the role of the advanced nurse practitioner. The work concludes with information and guidance about advance directives and advanced nurse practitioners.

The contents of this book are topical and pertinent to current advanced nursing practice issues. The main contributors are advanced nurse practitioners whose work and interests currently reflect the specialist issues they have chosen to write about. Each chapter concludes with key points that highlight the salient points raised, and direct the readers' thoughts to the issues of advanced practice for that topic.

It is hoped that this interesting and thought-provoking work will be of practical value to nurses as they push the boundaries of nursing forward and advance their own practice.

Ethics and advanced nursing practice

Karen Bartter

Introduction

There continues to be some debate about the title, function, role, responsibilities, sphere of practice, autonomy and accountability of the advanced nurse practitioner (ANP) (Davis, 1994; Davies and Hughes, 1995; Paniagua, 1995; Castledine and McGee, 1998; Hicks and Hennessy, 1998; Lillyman, 1998; Woods, 1999). However, as Elliott (1995) says:

> *the advanced nursing practitioner (ANP) is one of the most exciting and challenging concepts for British nursing . . .*

and the ANP is here, facing the challenges of and in advanced practice today.

The aim of this chapter is to revisit very briefly the concept of advanced practice in the literature, then to focus on and consider some of the potential areas of ethical conflict for the advanced nurse practitioner.

What is advanced practice?

What is advanced practice? What are its characteristics, and how is it achieved, measured and evaluated? In our world of compartmentalizing life, the nursing and medical professions have frequently looked to robust, testable measurements to 'prove' the validity of a given skill or criterion. But can this provide us with the blueprint of what an advanced nurse practitioner is?

The United Kingdom Central Council for Nursing, Midwifery and Health Visiting (UKCC), in *The Report of the Post-Registration Education and Practice Project* (UKCC, 1990), stated that:

> Only practitioners who have advanced their knowledge and skills through education and experience can exercise increased clinical discretion and accept greater professional responsibility through advanced practice.

In a later document, *The Future of Professional Practice – The Council's Standards for Education and Practice following Registration*, the UKCC identifies a need to 'adjust boundaries' for future advanced practice for this 'pioneering and developing new role responsive to changing needs' (UKCC, 1994). And although no exact, clear direction is given from the Council on specifics regarding qualifications or levels of knowledge and skills, aspects of the ANP role are identified. These include clinical practice, research, education and management, and the enriching of professional practice for the 'continuing development of the profession in the interests of patients, clients and the health service' (UKCC, 1994).

The characteristics of the ANP role are well cited in the literature (Davis, 1994; Davies and Hughes, 1995; Anon, 1996; Autar, 1996; Woods, 1998a, 1998b). Although each author may not cite exactly the same points in their definitions, the general thrust remains the same, which reflects the UKCC's views. As Paniagua (1995) succinctly puts it:

> Clearly, those in advanced nursing practice will need to demonstrate a considerable expertise above that of most specialist nurses.

Davies and Hughes (1995), however, argue that identifying the ANP by using a range of sub-roles does not do justice to the practitioner; nor does it clearly illuminate the broader picture of this multifaceted professional or the total contribution to health care the ANP can make. They do state that some of the functions identified in the sub-roles can be and are being very adequately performed in a small number of cases by specialist nurses who are not ANPs (as indeed there could conceivably be a few ANPs who do not fulfil their role parameters), but the totality of the ANP is more than a collection of sub-roles. Advanced practice is a method of thinking and approaching nursing challenges in a new way; encapsulating all the facets with an understanding of the broader context and a heightened sense of responsibility and accountability (Davies and Hughes, 1995).

When considering what is involved in the role of the ANP, Elliott (1995) suggests that there are two dimensions; the first is the scope of each individual ANP's practice, and the second is the level of the ANP's performance. Using this concept, it is within the scope that the characteristics of the role are included, and the level of performance is that which can identify the degree of advanced practice. Therefore, the appropriateness, complexity and accuracy of the assessment of a level of clinical practice are clearly difficult issues. The more advanced clinicians become, the greater the assessment problem; who is now able and practically credible to assess their performance? There is an argument that demonstration of advanced practice should be in the performance of skills with underpinning knowledge that the individual can critically think and reflect upon (Lillyman, 1998). Assessing all these criteria and how they interact and affect each other represents a complex task indeed, and one fraught with the potential for error.

Davis (1994) also discusses the difficulty in defining levels of nursing practice. He has produced a grid 'to enable all nurses to get a "feel" for what different levels of practice actually mean'. Here, elements of the sub-roles are referenced against 'outcome type' descriptions for Diploma, Bachelor, Master and Doctoral levels. This valuable guide for practitioners can most certainly be used to generate thought, reflection and discussion, and to assist in the identification of personal development needs for all levels of practitioners. For, as Davis states:

Being an 'expert' at Masters or Doctoral level in one element does not imply expertise in other elements.

The difficulty in clearly articulating the defining level and qualities of advanced practice seems to be felt by some ANPs themselves. Work by Hicks and Hennessy (1998) and Woods (1998a, 1998b, 1999) identifies that some ANPs have themselves experienced some role definition, role adjustment and scope of practice issues that cause them concern. Woods (1998b) cites four factors that were classifications of themes identified by ANPs as help or hindrances in their role:

1. Professional relationships
2. Individual practice
3. The clinical environment
4. Legislation.

Professional relationships, and how each practitioner faced the challenges of developing their own new professional role, was most frequently cited as having the potential for problems. This must clearly cover many possible situations. However, being accepted in a new role by old colleagues, and either being prevented from functioning in place of a medical officer when able to or being inappropriately used as a junior doctor are examples of potential stress and conflict (Kaufman, 1996; Woods, 1998b, 1999).

To assist practitioners in their new venture, there was some useful advice in the *Journal of Advanced Nursing* (Anon, 1996):

> *Advanced clinical nursing practice and expanded role function should be guided by a nursing model or emphasis. It should not be directed or dictated by physicians or a medical model.*

In this way, it will remain a distinct sphere of nursing.

Certainly a lot is expected of an ANP, such as a high degree of competence, a Masters degree and the ability to work closely with other health care team members (Castledine and McGee, 1998), as well as all the other role characteristics previously mentioned.

However, advanced practice, to follow the Gustalt theory (Curzon, 1985), is more than the sum of the parts. Advanced practice needs to be intrinsic and present throughout nursing skills: focusing, linking, fusing and encapsulating the total processes and, far more than these things, moving the nurse to truly holistic care – care of and with the client. This means taking into consideration the totality of the situation – the events of the present health care needs and characteristics, the social implications, a reflection into the reality of a particular client's past and future, and how these things might impact on the total health of the individual.

In the author's view, to aspire to advanced practice the nurse must operate on a different plane. Knowledge base and accurate skill ability must of course be excellent, and must continue to be developed and practised. However, it is also the *thinking* that sets the ANP apart. There must be depth and breadth of thinking, an intuitive cognition that transcends the normal realms of communication so the client *knows* that here is a nurse with that special indefinable something – something that instils in the client a knowledgeable peace that this nurse 'knows'. This view is well expressed by Davies and Hughes, who state that advanced nursing moves beyond roles to 'a way of thinking and viewing the world based on clinical knowledge' (Davies and Hughes, 1995). This involves not only high levels of knowledge and skills, but also facets of the individual nurse.

It must be identified here that some nurses have a spark of something – the obvious potential to be special in nursing. These people may not have undertaken any course but they should be encouraged to do so, so that under the right circumstances their special skill might be honed and the other characteristics of an identified ANP developed further. However, for most ANPs, as the literature generally identifies and agrees, in-depth knowledge, skills, some longevity of practice and advanced education input (preferably to Masters level) is essential to assist in the development of the individual to advanced practice (UKCC, 1990, 1994; Davis, 1994; Elliott, 1995; Anon, 1996; Castledine and McGee, 1998; Woods, 1998a; Courtenay, 2000).

Clearly, advanced practice is not a single milestone that is miraculously reached one day and then can be forgotten about; rather, it is a long and perhaps endless continuum. As practice, knowledge, cognition, skills etc. all continue to develop, so too does the potential for increased ethical dilemmas. What was once apparently simple and straightforward can now be, on deeper consideration, quite complex and convoluted, having the potential for personal mental anguish.

Ethical theories in the health care setting

Many excellent texts exist today to identify ethical theories, principles and codes, and their use within health care settings (Gillon, 1986; Beauchamp and Childress, 1989; Mackie, 1990; Billington, 1991; Tschudin, 1994; Singleton and McLaren, 1995; Thompson *et al.*, 1995; British Medical Association, 1996; McLean, 1996; Thiroux, 1998; Mason and McCall Smith, 1999; Palmer 1999), and it is not necessary to repeat these here. However, the application of some of the concepts many prove beneficial.

It is acknowledged that many of the ethical principles have been excellently and comprehensively addressed in other chapters in this book; however, their application is generally specific to the issues of each chapter. Here, the general principle and its application will be considered.

Frequently in texts ethical principles are cited singly or in pairs; in reality, they are frequently applied in larger groups. An example is that of paternalistic action in withholding information or a breach of fidelity being morally justified as acceptable by an individual who cites the principles of non-maleficence and beneficence owed to the client – that is, the professional perceives it as being in the client's best interests. In reality, the trade-off of principles to justify acts and/or omissions must be used extremely cautiously and with great consideration and reflection, lest practitioners find they are serving their own ends and not protecting or forwarding respect of personhood for the individual that they are charged to serve.

The hypothetical scenarios that follow the brief explanations of some of the principles are cited to provoke thought. Practitioners are invited to read, reflect and consider what the less than average, the average and the advanced professional would make of the situation, the action they would take or not take, and the justification they might put forward in each case.

Non-maleficence and beneficence

The two principles of non-maleficence and beneficence are well known and are frequently cited in the nursing texts. Non-maleficence could be considered as the oldest principle applied to humankind, coming as it does from the maxim *primum non nocere* – above all do no harm (Beauchamp and Childress, 1989). It is commonly held to be the basic principle owed by all of us to each other. Beneficence, the principle of promoting or benefiting the good of/for the individual (Singleton and McLaren, 1995), is considered to be central to nursing philosophy, application and care (UKCC, 1992a, 1992b). These two principles, both worthy of individual consideration by their own merits, will be considered together for the sake of expediency, as they are frequently traded off against each other to justify actions or omissions in health care situations.

Non-maleficence and beneficence can be seen as two ends of the same continuum, and are frequently applied in the same situation almost in the same breath. Every nursing intervention that causes distress, fear or pain breaches the principle of non-maleficence. The usual motivation for such a nursing intervention is to promote good for the patient or client; however, frequently nurses concentrate on the beneficent part of the act, and belittle or omit any consideration of non-maleficence and actually causing harm. Several examples of this occur in nursing each and every day – taking blood, giving injections, redressing wounds or injuries, and even pressure area care. In the case of children, the harm and distress caused by many of these types of interventions are considered and appropriate action taken, such as the application of topical local anaesthetics. Why is this not so for adults? Can there be a moral right in separating human subjects for the application of greater respect of non-maleficence when this is surely owed to all?

Consider which factors might influence the thinking of the less than average, the average and the advanced professional nurse when taking blood from a 5-year-old child, a 40-year-old adult and an 85-year-old adult.

It may be that some would argue that financial considerations apply, forwarding the view that older people can stand the pain to save the Health Service money. Think deeper into the application of ethics here. Consider the benefit and harm to each person in each situation, consider the non-maleficent view of affording no deliberate harm to anyone, and consider the general principle of human rights – not least to be offered the choice of pain control over saving costs to benefit oneself and others at a future time. However, the real-life dilemma of the cost of care cannot be disregarded. The expense to the NHS and the studious and appropriate application of scarce resources for a growing health care need encourage a utilitarian approach to the allocation of resources. The greatest good to the greatest number – the basic guiding tenet of the utilitarian theory (Beauchamp and Childress, 1989; Singleton and McLaren, 1995; Palmer, 1999) – in the application of health care resources would seem the best possible way to meet the needs of the majority. However, the general philosophy of the nursing disciplines (Tschudin, 1994; Thompson *et al.*, 1995; Clarke, 1996) and the professional guidance given to practitioners (UKCC, 1992a, 1992b, 1996) follow the doctrine of the deontological theory: duty, respect and responsibility towards, and the upholding of the primacy of, the individual. This juxtaposition of differing theories, each vying for equal recognition and compliance, with the nurse and client in the centre, is in itself a time bomb of potential dilemma for the practitioner. Add to this the nurse's requirement to 'justify public trust and confidence' in health care services and 'to uphold and enhance the good standing and reputations of the professions' (UKCC, 1992a), and it is little wonder that many a nurse feels pulled in several directions in trying the meet the needs of patients and clients.

Paternalism

When attempting to justify actions and in-actions in nursing and medicine, professionals frequently refer to the doctrine of the 'nurse/

doctor knows best'. This deference to paternalism may be a conscious or a subconscious mechanism to further the aim of the professional rather than truly attending to the best interests of the client.

Medical paternalism is the subject of extensive discussion in the literature and brief clarification of parts of the complexity of paternalism will be undertaken here. It must be clearly stated that paternalism is not considered to be an ethical principle, for what could be the moral or ethical reasoning or justification for actions and/or inactions that remove an individual's free will, deny autonomy and disrespect personhood?

There are many good definitions of paternalism; one such is that of Dworkin (1972), who states that paternalism is the:

> ... interference with a person's liberty of action justified by reasons referring exclusively to the welfare, good, happiness, needs, interests or values of the person coerced.

Beauchamp and Childress (1989) debate paternalism widely and clearly and, among other things, identify the argument of the superior professional knowledge, skills and training which oblige the professional to know about and to act in the patient's best interests. This point is also explored by Thiroux (1998) and Singleton and McLaren (1995). The point does hold some credence in that the professional, by dint of training and experience, is more knowledgeable. However, this knowledge, skill and experience concerns the condition/disease process and not the totality of the client as an individual, and as such, in this author's view, does not give any justification for accepting the use of any form of paternalism without deep and detailed consideration.

The authors cited also explore differing types of paternalism, such as 'weak' paternalism (where decisions are made for the best interests of an individual whose autonomy, for whatever reason, is severely diminished) and 'strong' paternalism (where a rational, competent individual capable of making an autonomous choice is limited or denied the freedom of that choice) (Beauchamp and Childress, 1989; Singleton and McLaren, 1995; Thiroux, 1998). It may be seen, then, that paternalism can be viewed as a continuum with weak (possibly in some cases justified) paternalism on one hand moving to strong paternalism at the other. Here strong paternalism manipulates and seeks to remove and deny the individual's autonomy. It may even, at worst, seek to further the ends of the professional at the expense of the client.

It is not correct to say that there is never any place for paternalism in health care. There are situations where its use clearly benefits the client and, rarely, where individuals autonomously hand over their right of self-determination to the professional. However, without exception, the ANP and all professionals who consciously use paternalism must examine their motivation and justifications very carefully. It behoves us all to look very closely at all our interactions with clients to examine them for signs of covert paternalism.

Consider the situation of a nurse working in general practice. A poorly dressed, vaguely unclean and generally unkempt middle-aged man, who smells of alcohol and has slight slurring of his speech, presents at a drop-in well man clinic. He is unknown to the practice, although he gives a home address that is within the catchment area. He states that he has recently moved to the area and is without a GP at present, but wishes to register with the practice for health care. He is reasonably articulate, but vague. The nurse feels sorry for the man and decides that, whilst she has asked and gained permission from him for some general health assessment checks, she will also undertake some others that she has not discussed with him. She also decides to advise him on diet, vitamin supplements and other things that will do him good. She strikes up a seemingly good conversation with the man, who is very obliging and thankful for her attention. Whilst examining him, the nurse notices an open wound on the man's upper arm and decides to take swabs, then clean, repair and dress the wound. This takes place without any discussion about her actions with the man. How do the principles of non-maleficence and beneficence, and the position of paternalism apply here? Was the nurse doing anything wrong?

Consent and veracity

Consent as a principle and a concept is widely talked about and discussed in the literature, both in other chapters of this book and in the texts previously cited, and extensive discussion is therefore not needed here. However, the principles of veracity – telling the truth – and self-determined autonomous choice are now explored a little further.

We will all find, if we examine our lives, actions and conversations closely, that in the normal course of everyday life we seldom uphold the principle of veracity absolutely. Whether in attempting to persuade children to comply, arranging surprises for family members or friends, explaining lateness or the failure to do something promised, or any number of other examples, human beings are less than totally truthful.

The truth can hurt, and thus omitting information, prevaricating or telling a 'white lie' in the 'people protection' mode – even to the level of deceitfulness – may be considered necessary. However, what reasons can be forwarded, how valid are the justifications, how clear is the moral conscience, and what principle trade-off has been made?

When any reduction in the application of absolute veracity is employed, for whatever reason, in the health care setting, the potential for loss of client autonomy and the exercising of personal choice is present.

Consider, for example, an ANP holding her own surgery who receives some test results confirming extensive cancer in a young client. The patient, a 35-year-old widow with two young children, comes for an arranged consultation that afternoon. How does the ANP proceed? Then consider the same ANP with the same test results, but this time the client is an 85-year-old woman who is fiercely independent, and has a fear of hospitals and a dread that she will die in one without any dignity. How does the ANP proceed in this case?

What are the justifications for the ANP's actions and in-actions in each case, what principles are applied, and, if each is dealt with differently, why is this?

Role development for the advanced nurse practitioner

What about the rights of the ANP? When considering issues of self-determination, autonomy and advocacy, the focus is primarily with the client – and rightly so. However, it should not be forgotten that the professional has rights as well as duties to others. Whilst examination of the personal rights of the ANP is not the issue here, some consideration will now be given to the practicalities of how ANP's might view their own professional self-determination, autonomy and advocacy in order to fulfil their role as an advanced practitioner as they see it.

Reference has been made earlier in this work to how some ANPs have experienced role adjustment difficulties and colleague acceptance friction (Hicks and Hennessy, 1998; Woods, 1998a, 1998b, 1999). These issues are explored further in a paper by Hunt (1999). Hunt also identifies findings from her research that demonstrate continuing confusion as to how community and hospital-based specialist nurses see themselves, and what specialist and advanced nurses actually are. Hunt also makes the point that specialist nurses, such as Florence Nightingale and Sister Dora, have always existed (Hunt, 1999). Such nurses have probably experienced problems in actualizing their ideals for their clients, just as ANPs might.

Another problem to consider here is how ANPs actually see themselves, how they and others consider the value of what they do, and how ANPs feel they are able to develop in, and on, their role.

Pullen believes that a huge part of the role of the ANP is that of an advocate. She says that the specialist practitioner's role moves her to be 'an advocate first, a nurse second' (Pullen, 1995). In order to act as an effective advocate, the ANP must be assertive and able to operate with self-determination and autonomy. However, the concept and reality of the ANP are still relatively new, and there are limited resources available to assist in their development once ANPs have taken up their initial post.

Gerry Kaufman, a Nurse Practitioner in West Yorkshire, has written about his role in a primary health care setting. He talks of the practicalities of his job and his views on some issues, such as advanced practice and autonomy and accountability. Kaufman also identifies some stresses of his job when he talks of concerns expressed by colleagues about nursing role erosion and the way that his role expansion might imply that current nursing practice in primary care could be substandard (Kaufman, 1996).

Role expansion and education

Some authors believe that role expansion and stretching the boundaries of nursing practice are intrinsic to the role of the ANP (Sutton and Smith, 1995; Kaufman, 1996). Yet in order to do these things the ANP would surely benefit from support and experience from others, as well as a finely developed sense of personal autonomy. To act with autonomy and as an advocate requires in-depth and thorough education and training, coupled with years of clinical experience, knowledge and skill. These things appear, to this author, to be cyclical and to have a degree of interdependence. However, ANPs also need to develop personal strategies to aid the furtherment of their role for the good of their clients and the profession as a whole. Elements of such a strategy might include reading relevant texts and keeping reflective diaries, but ANPs must each develop their own.

Valued and relevant texts in the subject area of their practice, including the reading and adding of pertinent articles to their knowledge store, is vital. The texts should also include legal and ethical sources, along with guidance from professional bodies, so that practice can be informed, guided and justified in all arenas.

Personal and professional reflective diaries help to demonstrate situations of past learning and importance and areas of current and future study; they act as a reference source and demonstrate the ongoing development of the individual. Confidentiality is, of course, of the utmost importance in any record keeping. This is vital in order to further the respect and protection of any and all clients, as well as recognizing the legal and professional obligations of the ANP and any nurse.

Considerations for personal role development

Good written, verbal and non-verbal communication is vital for clear and effective understanding between parties, and for good working relationships with colleagues. It is both useful and valuable for everyone to consider periodically how others might interpret what they say, write or do, in order to reduce ambiguity and the potential for causing confusion and offence.

Good communication includes the need to find time to talk to colleagues as well as clients. Many things change quickly, and all colleagues may not be aware of every advance and change. This communication, however, should not be solely work-related. All nurses, doctors and support staff, of whatever professional level, are also people with their own range of successes, problems and emotions.

Having a plan for a future project of development, or a target to work towards, helps to motivate good practice and a positive attitude to work. However, projects must be chosen carefully, as striving to achieve the impossible every day becomes soul destroying and disheartening.

Everyone needs a confidant with whom to share concerns, doubts and worries as well as achievements. This person should be chosen carefully, and it is important to remember the burden of confidentiality placed on them.

It benefits everyone to listen to the little warning voice in their head. In the presence of the strong feeling that something is not right, the whole situation should be re-examined, considering the reason for unease and determining possible actions – or in-action. We are all fallible human beings who can make mistakes, and it is better to admit to concern, anxiety or bafflement than to risk the life, health and respect of colleagues and clients. However, natural caution must not become a burden that hinders advanced practice.

Time for oneself is perhaps the most important need, and one that tends to be neglected. If practitioners are not revived with 'me time' as needed, they cannot expect to continue constantly to give of themselves to the same high level of commitment and skill.

Summary

This chapter has looked at facets of the role and characteristics of the advanced nurse practitioner. Consideration has been given to the application of some of the more commonly cited ethical principles, with regard to advanced nursing practice. This has been illustrated with some brief scenarios, and questions have been posed for the reader to consider. Finally, some ideas have been forwarded for consideration in the adaptation of a personal strategy for role development for each advanced nurse practitioner.

The future of advanced nursing practice is not mapped. Advanced nurse practitioners each have the potential to make of their role what they wish. However, they are all charged with the responsibility of developing nursing interactions and caring to the best level that fellow citizens could ever hope to experience.

Key points

- The advanced nurse practitioner is still a new and evolving nursing professional. Therefore the possibilities are limitless.
- Careful consideration must be made of ethical principles, and their use in health care interventions.
- Justifications of actions and in-actions in nursing care must be clear and well considered.
- The trade-off of principles that have the potential to reduce client autonomy and personhood should be avoided except in exceptional situations, and then only permitted as a last option and after careful consideration and reflection.
- Advanced nurse practitioners should develop their own strategy to assist them in their own personal and professional development.

References

Anon. (1996). The role and criteria of an advanced nurse practitioner. *Br. J. Nursing*, **5(5)**, 288–9.

Autar, R. (1996) Role of the nurse teacher in advanced nursing practice. *Br. J. Nursing*, **5(5)**, 298–301.

Beauchamp, T. and Childress, J. (1989). *Principles of Biomedical Ethics*, 3rd edn. Oxford University Press.

Billington, R. (1991). *Living Philosophy – An Introduction to Moral Thought*, 2nd edn. Routledge.

British Medical Association (1996). *Medical Ethics Today*. BMA.

Castledine, G. and McGee, P. (eds) (1998). *Advanced and Specialist Nursing Practice*. Blackwell Science.

Clarke, R. (1996). Midwifery autonomy and the code of professional conduct: an unethical combination. In: *Ethics and Midwifery: Issues in Contemporary Practice* (L. Frith, ed.), pp. 205–20. Butterworth-Heinemann.

Courtenay, M. (2000). *Advanced Nursing Skills: Principles and Practice*. Greenwich Medical Media.

Curzon, L. (1985). *Teaching in Further Education*, 3rd edn. Holt, Rinehart and Wilson.

Davies, B. and Hughes, A. (1995). Clarification of advanced nursing practice: characteristics and competencies. *Clin. Nurse Spec.*, **9(3)**, 156–66.

Davis, P. (1994). How to define levels of nursing practice. *Nursing Standard*, **8(26)**, 32–4.

Dworkin, R. (1972). In: *Moral Problems in Medicine: A Practical Coursebook* (M. Palmer), pp. 130–44. Lutterworth Press.

Elliott, P. (1995). The development of advanced nursing practice: 1. *Br. J. Nursing*, **4(11)**, 633–6.

Gillon, R. (1986). *Philosophical Medical Ethics*. John Wiley and Sons.

Hicks, C. and Hennessy, D. (1998). A task-based approach to defining the role of the nurse practitioner: the views of UK acute and primary sector nurses. *J. Adv. Nursing*, **29(3)**, 666–73.

Hunt, J. (1999). A specialist nurse: an identified professional role or a personal agenda? *J. Adv. Nursing*, **30(3)**, 704–12.

Kaufman, G. (1996). Nurse practitioners in general practice: an expanding role. *Nursing Standard*, **11(8)**, 44–7.

Lillyman, S. (1998). Assessing competence. In: *Advanced and Specialist Nursing Practice* (G. Castledine and P. McGee, eds), pp. 119–31. Blackwell Science.

Mackie, J. (1990). *Ethics: Inventing Right and Wrong*. Penguin Books.

Mason, J. and McCall Smith, R. (1999). *Law and Medical Ethics*, 5th edn. Butterworths.

McLean, S. (ed.) (1996). *Contemporary Issues in Law, Medicine and Ethics*. Dartmouth.

Palmer, M. (1999). *Moral Problems in Medicine: A Practical Coursebook*. Lutterworth Press.

Paniagua, H. (1995). The scope of advanced practice: action potential for practice nurses. *Br. J. Nursing*, **4(5)**, 269–74.

Pullen, F. (1995). Advocacy: a specialist practitioner role. *Br. J. Nursing*, **4(5)**, 275–8.

Singleton, J. and McLaren, S. (1995). *Ethical Foundations of Health Care*. Mosby.

Sutton, F. and Smith, C. (1995). Advanced nursing practice: new ideas, a new perspective. *J. Adv. Nursing*, **21(6)**, 1037–43.

Thiroux, J. (1998). *Ethics Theory and Practice*, 6th edn. Prentice Hall.

Thompson, I., Melia, K. and Boyd, K. (1995). *Nursing Ethics*. Churchill Livingstone.

Tschudin, V. (1994). *Deciding Ethically*. Bailliere Tindall.

United Kingdom Central Council (1990). *The Report of the Post-registration Education and Practice Project*. UKCC.

United Kingdom Central Council (1992a). *Code of Professional Conduct*. UKCC.

United Kingdom Central Council (1992b). *The Scope of Professional Practice*. UKCC.

United Kingdom Central Council (1994). *The Future of Professional Practice – The Council's Standards for Education and Practice following Registration*. UKCC.

United Kingdom Central Council (1996). *Guidelines for Professional Practice*. UKCC.

Woods, L. (1998a). Identifying the practice characteristics of advanced practitioners in acute and critical care settings. *Intens. Crit. Care Nursing*, **15**, 308–17.

Woods, L. (1998b). Implementing advanced practice: identifying the factors that facilitate and inhibit the process. *J. Clin. Nursing*, **7(3)**, 265–73.

Woods, L. (1999). The contingent nature of advanced nursing practice. *J. Adv. Nursing*, **30(1)**, 121–8.

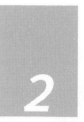

Contraception and the under 16s – legal and ethical implications for the advanced nurse practitioner

June Connolly

Introduction

Few groups in society excite as much public and policy concern as teenage mothers, and unfortunately the United Kingdom has the highest pregnancy rate amongst teenagers in Western Europe (The Social Exclusion Unit, 1999). In England there are nearly 90 000 conceptions a year to teenagers, approximately 7700 to girls below 16 years of age and 2200 to girls aged 14 or under, with roughly three-fifths (56 000) resulting in live births (The Social Exclusion Unit, 1999). In the 1970s the UK had similar teenage birth rates to other European countries; however, while other European countries achieved dramatic falls in the number of teenage pregnancies in the 1980s and 1990s, rates in the UK have remained static (The Social Exclusion Unit, 1999). There is no single explanation for the UK's high rates of teenage pregnancy (Family Policy Studies Centre, 1999). However, almost one in five young women and more than one in four young men have reported having sexual intercourse before their sixteenth birthday (FPA, 1997a), and a large-scale British survey discovered that approximately half of those having sex before the age of 16 years reported that they did not use any form of contraception (FPA, 1997b; Family Policy Studies Centre, 1999). Research has shown that most teenage mothers do not plan their pregnancies, resulting in half of all conceptions in under-16s and one-third of all teenage conceptions ending in abortion (Family Policy Studies Centre, 1999). The Health of the Nation strategy in England and Wales (DOH, 1992) identified the prevention of pregnancy in under-16s as a priority area, and commissioned a report. In its report to the Government on teenage pregnancies, The Social Exclusion Unit (1999) recommended that the Government needed an action plan to establish clear goals to halve the rate of conceptions among 18-year-olds in England by 2010, and to set a firmly established downward trend in the conception rates for under-16s by 2010.

There are two possible approaches that can be taken to reduce teenage conception: first, the moralistic approach, whereby young people are restricted so that they are unable to engage in sexual intercourse; and secondly, the pragmatic approach, whereby, young people are enabled to make an educated choice (Martin, 1996). The moralistic approach is very paternalistic, and removes the teenagers' right to choose and thus reduces their autonomy. In order to achieve the target set by The Social Exclusion Unit (1999) a more pragmatic approach is desired to enable teenagers to be self-determining. Therefore, young people require a service that is relevant to their needs, freely available, individualistic, informative, confidential, informal and accessible, and staffed by non-judgemental and sensitive health professionals. The advanced nurse practitioner (ANP), who holds a specialist qualification in family planning, is ideally placed in general practice to work in collaboration with the general practitioner in promoting such a service for young people, as nurses in practice are seen by many young people as easier to approach and talk to about sex and relationships than doctors (Wooton, 1995; Jeffree, 1997). Those in general practice have to walk a tightrope in the area of contraceptive advice for teenagers, which is a matter of topical interest and great concern for nurses and doctors and also for the general public and media. The author regularly comes into contact with issues concerning the under-16s and contraception within her family planning role as an ANP in general practice. This chapter will therefore examine the ethical and legal implications surrounding the issue of contraception and girls under the age of 16 years in general practice, as it is an issue that demonstrates how law and moral philosophy may intersect and interact with medicine and the extended future role of the ANP in general practice. The main areas that will be focused on are the law relating to contraceptive advice for girls under 16 years of age, consent, and confidentiality. This chapter does not attempt to provide answers or solutions regarding the ethical implications of this topic, but is merely intended to promote a deeper understanding of the issues raised.

Legal and ethical implications

The law

Before considering issues of consent and confidentiality, it is important to examine the legal aspects relating to the law and sexual intercourse in the under-16s. In England, Wales and Scotland, a young woman must be 16 years of age before she can consent to sexual intercourse; in Northern Ireland she has to be 17 (Brook Advisory Centres, 1996). Throughout the UK, any male over the age of criminal responsibility (i.e.10 years old) who has unlawful sexual intercourse with a girl under the age of consent is breaking the law. If a young woman under 16 years of age does have sexual intercourse, she is not committing an offence; it is the male partner who commits the offence (Brook Advisory Centres, 1996; FPA, 1997c). Under Section 5 of the Sexual Offences Act (England and Wales) 1956, it is an absolute offence (no defence of mistaking the age of the girl is allowed) for a male to have unlawful sexual intercourse with a girl under 13 years of age. However, under Section 6 of the same Act it is a less serious offence for a male to have sexual intercourse with a girl between the ages of 13 and 16 (Mason and McCall Smith, 1991; Brook Advisory Centre, 1996; FPA, 1997c). Various defences are available to the male in these circumstances:

1. If the male is under 24 and has not been previously charged with a similar offence, and believes the girl to be 16 or over.
2. That the man justifiably believes himself married to the girl (whilst the marriage is not valid). This could arise when the marriage takes place in another country with a lower age of legal marriage (FPA, 1997c).

Considering the laws relating to the age of consent to sexual intercourse poses the question of whether the practitioner (doctor/ANP), in prescribing or giving contraceptive advice to girls under 16, could be seen as an accessory to crime. In law, a person is liable as an accessory if he or she aids, abets, counsels or procures the commission of a crime (Kennedy, 1996). It is presumed to be very unlikely that a doctor or ANP would encourage sexual intercourse in girls under 16, and even rarer that they would incite or conspire with her male partner to do so. The conscience of the medical profession and also the courts of law have been torn apart wondering whether to prescribe contraceptive pills to girls under the age of 16 years (Mason and McCall-Smith, 1991).

This dilemma has been increased by morality campaigners and Family Law Action groups, who continue to accuse the medical profession of 'handing out pills' with no questions asked and without parental knowledge, and they continually call for clinics to be banned from giving contraception to girls under 16 years (Doughty, 1998). It is important to note that most young girls seek contraceptive advice only after they have become sexually active, and usually following unprotected sex (Andrews, 1997). However, family campaigners reason that the law is being abandoned because increasing numbers of girls under 16 have sex illegally but legal actions against men and teenage boys are not rising accordingly (Hall, 1998). It is interesting that the experience of many doctors who examine the 'victim' of the offence is that she is usually candid, unrepentant and unaffected by the intervention of the law (Mason and McCall-Smith, 1991).

Many of the statements made by morality campaigners appear to be paternalistic, and involve either limiting or denying freedom of choice in health care decisions regarding contraception for girls under 16 years. Young girls are growing up in a society that is beginning to challenge the notion that sex is a male prerogative and recognize that females too are capable of sexual desires (Jackson, 1982) and are attempting to take control of their lives and sexuality. Numerous rules and conventions exist in society to define sex as the preserve of adults (e.g. the age of consent laws), and these are outward signs of the taboo surrounding minors and sex and to even question them is to invite a hostile response from conservative campaigners against sexual 'permissiveness' (Jackson, 1982). Many adults tend to underestimate the maturity of minors (under-16s), and tend to forget that minors, according to the 1959 Declaration of Rights of the Child, are as entitled as adults to have their needs met and to liberty rights (Black, 1991).

Consent

With reference to the law and rights, Section 8 of the omnibus Family Law Reform Act declared that consent to medical treatment could be given by a minor of 16 years of age, and in such cases parental consent was not needed (MDU, 1996). Section 8.3 of the same Act appeared to consider that consent for under-16s could be valid in certain cases, such as confidential access to contraception (Kessel, 1993). This view of under-16s' legal rights was strengthened in Gillick *v.* West Norfolk & Wisbech Area Health Authority (1985). The issue of patient competence was at the centre of the House of Lords ruling, in deciding that in many cases girls under 16 years of age would be able to give consent to contraceptive treatment and advice. The court held that the crucial factor was the individual client's ability to understand, in broad terms, the nature and purpose of what was proposed (Stauch, 1998). Since the 1985 House of Lords ruling on the Gillick case, 'competent' people under 16 are legally able to consent, in certain circumstances, to medical treatment and contraceptive advice without parental consent (Winfield, 1997). This means that doctors and nurses can provide contraceptive advice and supplies for minors without parental consent, as long as the doctor/ANP is satisfied that the minor fulfils the criteria set out by Lord Fraser, in the following circumstances (Dyer, 1985; MDU, 1996):

● The girl can understand the doctor's advice (although under 16)
● She cannot be persuaded to inform, or allow the doctor to inform, her parents that she is seeking contraceptive advice
● She is likely to have sexual intercourse with or without contraception
● Unless she receives contraceptive advice it is likely that her health will suffer, mentally/physically or both
● It is in the girl's best interests to receive contraceptive advice, treatment or both without parental consent.

Therefore, if a doctor advises or prescribes contraceptives for a girl under 16 in good faith, an action in the criminal court for aiding and abetting in the commission of unlawful sexual intercourse would be unsuccessful (Martin, 1996). The Children's Act (1989) supports the approach taken by the House of Lords in the Gillick case – that the courts should ascertain the child's feelings and wishes, considered in the light of her age and understanding (Charles-Edwards, 1991). The current law specifically relates to doctors' actions, and this may cause a dilemma for ANPs in their future autonomous role in providing contraceptive services to minors. ANPs may well be in a position where they have to decide if a young girl under 16 has sufficient understanding to make an autonomous decision regarding contraceptive services.

The ethical dilemma

It has been reported that the majority of under-age girls who seek contraception are already aware that they are at risk of pregnancy and that their partner is committing a criminal offence, and also that they make an autonomous decision to ask for contraceptive care from their doctor or nurse and deserve to be treated with respect for the young adults they have shown themselves to be (Winfield, 1997). Practitioners themselves may not agree with the principles of prescribing contraceptives to girls under 16 years of age, and discover that their legal and moral accountability are in conflict, but they are bound by their Code of Professional Conduct (UKCC, 1992) to respect choices made by clients and remain non-judgemental. Respect for an individual requires that each person must be treated as unique and as an equal to every other person (Edwards, 1997). When faced with an ethical dilemma, the practitioner has to decide which of the possible options is the right action to take and how the choice of this action over any other can be justified. Actions can then be explained by demonstrating the ethical principles that justify them (Fletcher *et al.*, 1995). One way of trying to decide if an action is the right thing to do or not is to examine the consequences of performing that action and, in relation to contraceptive provision for under-16s, the consequences for the girl if the action is not performed. The right to contraception being denied could result in an unwanted pregnancy for the young girl. However, it could also be argued that by having sexual intercourse at an early age the risk of sexually transmitted disease and cervical cancer is increased. Then there is the issue that the government wishes to reduce conceptions in under-16s, as it has been shown that the costs of providing contraceptive and counselling services are far less than the health and social costs of unplanned pregnancy. For the ANP who is bound by a duty of care and who wishes to act with beneficence and non-maleficence, ethical and legal principles are in conflict; in this situation, respect for the autonomy of the rational young girl takes precedence (Singleton and McLaren, 1995).

Respecting autonomy

Medical practitioners have a duty of care to ensure that they respect the choices young girls make concerning their own lives, as trust and respect for the autonomy of individuals, it has been argued, are the vital foundation of the therapeutic relationship (Singleton and McLaren, 1995). There is a temptation for the practitioner, when dealing with young girls under 16, to override their autonomy and become paternalistic. However, individuals must be free to make up their own minds about what is right and wrong if they are to be morally responsible for what they do (Kant, 1785). It is morally essential to show 'respect for persons' by ensuring that they are able to make as many informed decisions and be as self-determining as possible (Tschudin, 1993). Recognizing a client's right to choose is clearly outlined in clauses 1 and 5 of the *Code of Professional Conduct for Nurses, Midwives and Health Visitors* (UKCC, 1992). In clause 5 of the code, the professional's role in promoting client independence is outlined. This means that it is important to discuss any proposed treatment or care with clients to enable clients to make an informed choice and decide what is in their own best interests (UKCC, 1996). The legal provision of contraceptive services in the UK requires practitioners to obtain consent to ensure that such care is not unwanted and is acceptable to the individual concerned (Martin, 1996). For consent to be valid, and for treatment to be lawful, three conditions must be satisfied: the patient must be competent (or 'have capacity'); there must be no duress or undue influence; and the client must be suitably informed about the nature of the proposed treatment (Stauch, 1998). To be able to consent, girls under 16 should not only understand the nature of the proposed treatment, but also have full understanding and appreciation of the consequences of the treatment, and of its failure (MDU, 1996).

In English law, children under 16 may refuse to give consent to medical treatment if the child concerned is of sufficient understanding to make an informed choice (Children's Act, 1989). Both the Children's Act (1989) and the Gillick judgement imply that the doctor must decide whether the young girl is competent. This puts an onus on the doctor, as no guidance or clarification of competence is offered. It also presumes that all doctors and nurses are sagacious, which they are not (Charles-Edwards, 1991), and the assumption that the 'doctor knows best' violates the young person's autonomy. Gillick competence has become the accepted measure for girls under 16 to be able to give consent to contraceptive treatment and advice, but how is 'competence' defined in young girls under 16? Criteria defining the degree of intelligence and understanding needed to be competent have not been clearly declared in English law (Fletcher *et al.*, 1995), and no specific test for competence exists. In law and medicine, standards of competence tend to feature mental skills or capacities closely connected to the attributes of autonomous persons, such as cognitive skills and independence of judgement (Beauchamp and Childress, 1994). Standards for competence in clinical medicine have been clustered around the various abilities to understand and process information, and to reason about the consequences of one's actions (Beauchamp and Childress, 1994). Therefore, in a biomedical context a person has generally been viewed competent if able to understand medical treatment or advice. The level of understanding and ability to reason required is not that of a professor of moral philosophy; it is the level that can be achieved by most adults and 14-year-olds (Charles-Edwards, 1991). Research conducted by Weithorn and Campbell (1982) into child development has demonstrated that most 14-year-olds have the same level of competence to make decisions such as consent to treatment as most adults. Piaget and Inhelder (1958) also discovered that children from the age of 12 years entered into the stage of 'formal operations', and were able to reason about hypothetical abstract situations, review possibilities, think about their thoughts, and see problems from others' perspectives.

The ANP cannot assume that because a young girl presents herself for treatment, consent has been given (Dimond, 1995). Consent to treatment can be given in various ways – written, verbal (expressed consent) or even a gesture (implied consent) (Dimond 1995) – and all of these forms of consent are valid in law, although written consent provides more 'solid' evidence (Hewston, 1994; Martin, 1996; Power, 1997). The client's informed consent to treatment can only be given if she has received adequate information on which to base her decision. In the case of contraceptive care, this means that the practitioner must fully inform the young girl about the range of contraceptives available and give details on their mode of action, efficacy and side-effects – both adverse and beneficial (Winfield, 1997) – without bias. If the practitioner fails to give this information to the girl, then the practitioner could be viewed as negligent. The practitioner must explain the facts of treatment to the girl using language that she is able to understand, as 'informed consent' without understanding is worthless (Fletcher *et al.*, 1995).

Care must be taken to ensure that the ANP does not make any assumptions regarding the patient's knowledge of even the most basic aspects of care or treatment (UKCC, 1996). However, it is worth noting that in the case of Sidaway *v.* Bethlem Royal Hospital Governors in 1985 it was claimed that inadequate information about the potential risks from surgery, which left the patient paralysed, had not been given before the operation. Although this was proved, Sidaway's case was lost at trial, at appeal and in the Lords on the basis that the surgeon had adhered to accepted practice in accordance with the Bolam test. This means that the amount of detail required to ensure valid consent is the amount that a responsible body of practitioners would provide in the same circumstances (Forshaw, 1995; Martin, 1996). This poses the question, if it were an ANP on trial in similar circumstances, would he or she be judged by other ANPs or similar nursing professionals, or would the 'responsible body of practitioners' passing judgement be doctors? ANPs as registered nurses are accountable for their own actions and answerable to the law and their Code of Professional Conduct (UKCC, 1992); however, to maintain a valid defence perhaps it would be advisable for ANPs to ensure that protocols are used in their particular area of expertise.

Accountability

Any person who professes to have a special skill or training (such as an ANP) upon which others rely will be in a position of responsibility and may therefore be held legally accountable for his or her actions (Fletcher *et al.*, 1995). ANPs must ensure that they are proficient and knowledgeable regarding current practices concerning contraceptive care in order to divulge correct and current information concerning the whole range of contraceptives to a young girl. The *Guidelines for Professional Practice* (UKCC, 1996) suggest that failure to provide adequate information could lead to a charge of battery in law; if it can be proved that inadequate information was given, consent may be invalid (Forshaw, 1995). Failure to inform patients adequately and to confirm their understanding of the information given when obtaining their consent could be construed as a failure to fulfil the duty of care adequately, and therefore result in a negligent action by the ANP (Dimond, 1997). However, if the practitioner is able to demonstrate, by contemporaneous records, that Gillick principle requirements were satisfied, the consent of the girl under 16 would be accepted by the law as valid for contraceptive services (Martin, 1996). If there is valid consent, then there is no tort of battery. In order to maintain the validity of consent, it must be given without fraud (Dimond, 1995). Therefore, ANPs must ensure that, where they are undertaking a procedure that may normally be thought of as being carried out by a doctor, patients do not assume that they are general medical practitioners (Friend, 1996). They must inform patient of their status to maintain the validity of consent. As long as the rules are obeyed and duty is fulfilled, no wrong can be done, according to deontologists (Naidoo and Willis, 1994).

Confidentiality

A girl under 16 years of age seeking contraceptive advice is often going to be as much concerned about her parents hearing of her request as about whether she has the capacity to give valid consent to treatment. This raises the question of whether or not a doctor or nurse is obliged to respect and observe the girl's confidentiality (Fletcher *et al.*, 1995). Young girls are often adamant that parents must not find out about their sexual activity. James (1988) reports that a young girl's parents have no absolute right in law to be informed of her intention to seek contraceptive advice if she is under 16. A doctor or nurse should not disclose the information to anyone else, but should encourage the young girl to inform her parents or guardian that she is seeking contraceptive advice or treatment, and should offer advice on ways of broaching such discussions. If the young girl does not wish the information to be disclosed, the doctor is still able to give contraceptive advice or treatment. Doctors may not override the wishes of the young girl except in exceptional circumstances (Brook Advisory Centres, 1996), and this principle should be the same for the ANP.

Confidentiality is a moral, legal and professional duty. Preserving confidentiality can be justified on the consequential grounds that it will maximize benefits to the young girl, who will be able openly to divulge to the doctor/ANP information that is vital to her treatment and other aspects of care (Singleton and McLaren, 1995). Confidentiality is then justified morally, in that the best possible outcomes in care are achieved for the individual; it can also be justified in a duty-based framework by protection. The basis for the legal duty arises from both the nurse's contract of employment, which should contain a requirement of confidentiality (either implied or expressed), and the common law duty of confidence relating to the professional relationship between nurse and patient (Pennels, 1998). Professionally, Clause 10 of the *Code of Professional Conduct* (UKCC, 1992) requires nurses to:

> ... *protect all confidential information concerning patients and clients obtained in the course of professional practice and make disclosures only with consent, where ... you can justify disclosure in the wider public interest ...*

Here, an obligation of confidentiality derives from a promise or undertaking that the information will not be divulged to a third party (Cain, 1998).

The UKCC Advisory Paper *Confidentiality* (1987), which has since been superseded by the *Guidelines for Professional Practice* (UKCC, 1996), believes that the focal word in the debate of confidentiality, is 'TRUST' (in capital letters). To trust another person with private and personal information about yourself is a significant matter (Cain, 1998).

Trust, according to Beauchamp and Childress (1994), is a confident belief in and reliance upon the ability and moral character of another person, and entails a confidence that another will act with the right motives in accord with moral norms. Trust also means that we have confidence in our ability to help (Tschudin, 1992). However, a practitioner's perceived lack of trustworthiness may be the primary reason for a young girl under 16 making a decision to consult another doctor/ANP on matters concerning contraceptive care. Anyone can consult another GP for contraceptive advice and treatment if they do not wish to consult their own GP. If a young girl under 16 is receiving contraceptive advice or treatment from another doctor or family planning clinic, the young girl's own GP does not legally have to be informed. However, the doctor/ANP should explain to the young girl that it is in her best medical interest for her own GP to be informed. If the young girl is assured that the information will be treated in confidence, it is unlikely that she will refuse. However, if she does refuse, then her decision must be respected (Brook Advisory Centres, 1996). By implication, the House of Lords judgement reinforced the principle that a girl under 16 has a right to seek treatment in confidence. In relation to the provision of contraception for girls under 16, the British Medical Association's (1994) guidance to GPs emphasized that the duty of confidentiality owed to a person under 16 is as great as the duty owed to any other person.

Confidentiality is a person's right, and therefore keeping confidentiality is 'doing good' (Tschudin, 1993). Keeping a confidence could also be doing others harm, and if this is the case confidentiality should not be upheld. If a doctor or nurse believes that a young girl under 16 seeking contraceptive advice and advice on sexual matters is being exploited, coerced or abused, the practitioner should counsel the young person with a view to persuading her to allow confidentiality to be relaxed. If the patient expresses that she does not want this, and the practitioner believes that she (or even another minor) continues to be at risk, the practitioner may have to break confidentiality (Brook Advisory Centres, 1996). This should not be done without informing the patient first.

There are four situations in which confidential information can be disclosed (UKCC, 1996; Pennels, 1998):

1. Disclosure by consent
2. Disclosure by required law
3. Disclosure in the public interest
4. Disclosure required by the police.

The disclosures most relevant to contraceptive cases would be disclosure by consent and disclosure required by law. Disclosure by consent includes both implied and expressed consent to disclose information. Consent must always be voluntary and meaningful. Implied consent arises most frequently when health professionals need to share relevant confidential information concerning the patient – in the case of contraceptive services for the young girl, the doctor and nurse will need to share information concerning treatments and medical contraindications, for example, to the contraceptive pill. What is important is that the young girl understands that some information may be made available to others involved in the delivery of her care (UKCC, 1996). Consent for disclosure should never be presumed, and the client must know with whom the information will be shared (UKCC, 1996).

Disclosure required by law is controlled by statute, which obliges nurses and health professionals either to disclose or withhold information – for example, in the case of a young girl being sexually abused or forced into prostitution against her will. Also, the Abortion Act 1967 requires details of terminations to be reported to the Department of Health.

In deciding whether to disclose information, the practitioner's overriding consideration must always be what is in the best interests of the young person (MDU, 1997). From both legal and moral perspectives, the rationales for maintaining the confidentiality of information relating to individuals are extremely powerful and compelling. Strong justifications must be made for breaking this duty, which should only occur in exceptional situations (Singleton and McLaren, (1995). If a professional thinks that disclosure of confidential information is morally justified or perhaps mandatory in a particular circumstance, then they should bear the burden of proof. Although this approach requires a balancing of conflicting duties, it also demonstrates a structure of moral reasoning and justification (Beauchamp and Childress, 1994).

Summary

In examining the ethical and legal implications surrounding the issues of the law, consent and confidentiality in relation to contraception in girls under 16 years, this chapter has raised many moral and ethical dilemmas. Most aspects of nursing have ethical and moral dimensions, but these are particularly difficult to tackle in family planning in relation to girls under 16 years of age, due to social values and expectations regarding what is acceptable and what is 'normal' behaviour in society. It is therefore essential that ANPs familiarize themselves with the law and ethics regarding this topic, so that they are able to justify any actions taken in that extended role. These issues will impinge more directly on ANPs' future practice as responsibilities increasingly cut across traditional boundaries between medicine and nursing.

Key points

- The UK has the highest teenage pregnancy rate in Western Europe, with nearly 90 000 conceptions a year to teenagers in England.
- Accessible, acceptable and reliable contraception is a valuable key to reducing the unplanned teenage pregnancy rate.
- Confidentiality is of paramount importance in all areas of health care, particularly in relation to sexual health matters.
- The law regarding sex and under-age teenagers is complex, and advanced nurse practitioners must be aware of the law relating to their practice in this area.
- Many ethical issues influence views on the sexual activities of teenagers, but those who seek contraception services deserve to be treated with respect as the young and responsible adults they have shown themselves to be.
- Advanced nurse practitioners are best placed to ensure valid informed consent in relation to contraception services and teenagers.

References

Andrews, G. (1997). Contraceptive advice – helping women make an informed choice. *Practice Nurse*, **14(3)**, 185–90.
Beauchamp, T. T. and Childress, J. F. (1994). *Principles of Biomedical Ethics*, 4th edn. Oxford University Press.
Black, D. (1991). The UN Convention on the Rights of the Child. *Briefings Med. Ethics*, **9**, 1–4.

British Medical Association (1994). *Confidentiality and People Under 16. Guidance Issued by the BMA, GMS, FDA & RCGP.* BMA.

Brook Advisory Centres (1996). *What Should I Do?* Brook Advisory Centres.

Cain, P. (1998). The limits of confidentiality. *Nursing Ethics,* **5(2)**, 158–65.

Charles-Edwards, I. (1991). Who decides? *Paed. Nursing,* **Dec.,** 6–8.

Department of Health (1992). *The Health of The Nation.* HMSO.

Dimond, B. (1995). *Legal Aspects of Nursing,* 2nd edn. Prentice Hall.

Dimond, B. (1997). *Legal Aspects of Care in the Community.* Macmillan Press Ltd.

Doughty, S. (1998). One in Ten Girls On Pill By 15. Newsprint, February 1998. Brook Advisory Centres.

Dyer, C. (1985). The Gillick judgement: contraceptives and the under 16s: House of Lords ruling. *Br. Med. J.,* **291**, 1208–9.

Edwards, M. (1997). Patient autonomy. *Practice Nurse,* **14(3)**, 206–8.

Family Policy Studies Centre (1999). Teenage pregnancy and the family. *Family Briefing Paper 9.* Family Policy Studies Centre.

Family Planning Association (1997a). *Young people; Sexual Attitudes & Behaviour,* Fact Sheet No. 9. CES.

Family Planning Association (1997b). *Teenage Pregnancy,* Fact Sheet No. 8. CES.

Family Planning Association (1997c). *The Law on Sex,* Fact Sheet No. 11. CES.

Fletcher, N., Holt, J., Brazier, M. and Haris, J. (1995). *Ethics, Law and Nursing.* Manchester University Press.

Forshaw, S. (1995). Treatment without consent. *Nursing Times,* **91(1)**, 27–9.

Friend, B. (1996). Risky business? *Nursing Times,* **92(30)**, 26–7.

Hall, C. (1998). Fall in Sex Crime Points to Crisis in Consent Law. Newsprint, February 1998. Brook Advisory Centres.

Hewston, G. (1994). Ignorance is not bliss. Informed consent. *Br. J. Theatre Nursing,* **4(9)**, 14–16.

Jackson, S. (1982). *Childhood and Sexuality.* Basil Blackwell.

James, C. (1988). Contraceptive practice: Some medico-legal questions answered. *J. Med. Defence Union,* **Summer**, 30–31.

Jeffree, P. (ed.) (1997). Sex is the word. *Practice Nurse,* **13(4)**, 185.

Kant, I. (1785). *Groundwork of The Metaphysics of Morals* (trans. H. J. Paton, 1948, as *The Moral Law*). Hutchinson.

Kennedy, I. (1996). *Treat Me Right – Essays in Medical Law and Ethics.* Clarendon Press.

Kessel, R. (1993). In the UK children can't just say No. *Hastings Centre Report,* **Mar/Apr,** 20–21.

Martin, J. (1996). Contraception and the under-16s: the legal issues. *Nat. Assoc. Nurses Contraception Sexual Health J.,* **32,** 106–10.

Mason, J. K. and McCall Smith, R. A. (1991). *Law and Medical Ethics,* 3rd edn. Butterworths.

Medical Defence Union (1996). *Consent to Treatment.* MDU.

Medical Defence Union (1997). *Confidentiality.* MDU.

Naidoo, J. and Willis, J. (1994). *Health Promotion: Foundations for Practice.* Balliere Tindall.

Pennels, C. J. (1998). Confidentiality. *Prof. Nurse*, **13**(7), 437–8.

Piaget, J. and Inhelder, B. (1958). *The Growth of Logical Thinking from Childhood to Adolescence*. Routledge & Kegan Paul.

Power, K. J. (1997). The legal and ethical implications of consent to nursing procedures. *Br. J. Nursing*, **6**(15), 885–7.

Singleton, J. and McLaren, S. (1995). *Ethical Foundations of Health Care Responsibilities in Decision Making*. Mosby.

Stauch, M. (1998). Consent in medical law. *Br. J. Nursing*, **7**(2), 84.

The Social Exclusion Unit (1999). *Teenage Pregnancy*. The Stationery Office.

Tschudin, V. (1992). *Ethics In Nursing. The Caring Relationship*, 2nd edn. Butterworth-Heinemann.

Tschudin, V. (ed.) (1993). *Ethics, Nurses and Patients*. Scutari Press.

United Kingdom Central Council (1987). *Confidentiality*. UKCC.

United Kingdom Central Council (1992). *Code of Professional Conduct*. UKCC.

United Kingdom Central Council (1996). *Guidelines for Professional Practice*. UKCC.

Weithorn, L. A. and Campbell, S. B. (1982). The competency of children and adolescents to make informed treatment decisions. *Child Dev.*, **53**, 1589–98.

Winfield, J. (1997). Let's talk about sex. *Practice Nurse*, **13**(6), 328–32.

Wooton, G. (1995). *The Nurse's Role in the Provision of Emergency Contraception*. RCOG Faculty of Family Planning & Reproductive Care.

3 The abortion issue and advanced nursing practice

Karen Harley

Introduction

The abortion issue is a popular topic for dissemination in ethical debates; it is a highly emotive, divisive and complex issue. From the outset, there appears to be no compromise in a polarized argument. Theoretical moral questions inherent in the abortion debate cannot be solved by factual evidence, producing deadlock (Seedhouse and Lovett, 1992). It is therefore important to recognize that the issue must be discussed as a two-sided argument, which contains and respects the attitudes, opinions and beliefs from both sides of the divide. The debate must include a fair representation of all of the arguments involved from all points along a spectrum of extremes. Consensus may not be reached, but the confusion, controversy and bitter arguments fought over the issue may become less polarized and more amenable to reason. The landmark work of Dworkin (1993) is invaluable in comprehending the nature of the debate. Dworkin challenges the standard view of the abortion argument and identifies intellectual confusion to reach a settlement that everyone can accept with full self-respect intact.

Ethical issues

Ethical analysis of abortion is often presented in terms of identifying the moral dilemmas involved. Each alternative choice can be justified by principles or moral rules (Benjamin and Curtis, 1992), none of which may be wholly satisfactory (Rumbold, 1986). Generally the debate is between 'pro-choice' and anti-abortion groups, 'pro-life', and it involves the conflict and reveals the complexities between two basic principles; the principle of individual freedom that represents the argument for bodily self-determination, and the principle of the value or sanctity of life (Thiroux, 1995). This in turn leads to a discussion of the philosophical issues involved. These may include the definition of personhood and clarification of when human life begins, and at what point it is to be valued and protected. The distinction between humans and persons, as Clarke (1999) asserts, is the divisive factor in the ethical debate on abortion.

From time immemorial, unplanned conceptions have ended in abortion. Despite recent advances in contraception, for which women usually take responsibility, none is 100 per cent effective; contraception fails, and fails to be used effectively. In 1999, 183 200 abortions were performed in England and Wales (provisional figure; Office of National Statistics, 2000). Worldwide, the World Health Organization (WHO) has calculated that approximately 50 million pregnancies are terminated by abortion each year (Loudon *et al.*, 1995). Abortion is and will continue to be a necessary component of women's reproductive health care. Often the first point of contact for women with unplanned pregnancies takes place in the primary health care setting. Whatever health care workers' personal beliefs regarding the abortion issue, they must be aware of their feelings (Dyson and White, 1999); there is a moral and professional responsibility either to provide unbiased information and support, or to refer a woman to a professional who can supply such information. It is important to realize that for most women an unplanned, unwanted pregnancy is an emotionally devastating experience, and the decision to abort is not taken lightly. It is often a decision that can have a profound effect on the women and on their entire lives (Davies, 1991).

An advanced practitioner working in primary health care will undoubtedly be involved in contentious ethical issues. While direct involvement in the ethical dimension surrounding abortion may be relatively uncommon, abortion and perhaps euthanasia are very popular topics in ethical debates given the moral controversy involved. Greater ethical understanding is therefore a necessary component in the knowledge base of advanced nurse practitioners (ANPs). Nurses who wish to expand their practice to provide a holistic comprehensive nursing service may be involved in ethical reasoning previously felt to be within the medical province. Traditionally, nurses are associated with physical and devoted bedside care. With the advent of advanced nursing practice, this stereotypical image of the nurse is no longer the case. The last decade has witnessed unprecedented changes in our health care system, and many nurses have seized the opportunity to develop, expand and improve services for their clients via improved clinical knowledge and the development of expertise. Advanced nursing practice will provide an innovative holistic service focusing on and optimizing client care within a nursing framework that is complementary to medicine. ANPs will therefore require a deeper understanding of ethical dilemmas to increase their capacity for advanced clinical reasoning (Fryer, 1995), a necessary competency of the ANP. Although this is applied here to the abortion issue, it may well be equally applicable to numerous ethical issues in health care.

Arguably, *The Scope of Professional Practice* (UKCC, 1992) provided the most influence in expanding the clinical practice of nurses. The document offered unparalleled opportunities for nurses to develop and expand their clinical role to become autonomous flexible practitioners, responding to the needs of their clients (Autar, 1996). In the community setting, *The Scope of Professional Practice* (UKCC, 1992) has been influential in providing the foundations for nurse-led clinics in general practice. Nurse-led family planning clinics are becoming more commonplace in the community. Nurses who undertake this advanced role in family planning services will certainly come into contact with women who became pregnant and did not plan to do so. Whilst many unplanned pregnancies become a happy event, others, for a number of reasons, end in termination. Counselling women who experience an unwanted pregnancy is perhaps one of the most challenging consultations a practitioner undertakes. An informed decision can only be made when the woman receives enough information on the different options available. The client seeking abortion requires good standards of practice in referral procedures to prevent contradictory advice and delays. The ANP can provide practical information regarding, for example, local provision and costs. Together with this practical knowledge, the ANP requires ethical knowledge to provide insight into this moral and ethically charged situation.

A major responsibility of ANPs is to empower their clients (Snyder and Mirr, 1995). Empowerment is a fundamental ethic (Rodwell, 1996), and should be uppermost on the agenda in a nurse-led family planning service, as the practitioner empowers clients to make informed choices in taking responsibility for their own bodies. Advocacy and autonomy are important related issues. Advocacy is an integral part of caring, and is therefore essential (Adams *et al.*, 1997). Moreover, caring is a function of expert nurses, and therefore of a nurse-led service. Client advocacy is claimed as the new role of the professional nurse (Malik, 1997), and is essential to a holistic model of advanced practice. Patient autonomy is defined as the potential for self-determination, and occurs when patients have the necessary information to consider treatment that is consistent with their beliefs and wishes (Edwards, 1997) – as, for example, when a woman experiences an unplanned pregnancy. Extending the nurse's role in areas such as a nurse-led family planning clinic increases autonomy and empowerment. The scenario of the client requesting an abortion and being advised, against her wishes, to continue the pregnancy, or being subjected to a deliberate delay in referral that may compromise safe, early abortion is unethical (BMA, 1998), and would become less commonplace.

Philosophical theories

The arguments surrounding abortion are more concerned with attitudes, values, opinions and beliefs, covering a diversity of moral opinion, in contrast to non-abstract aspects of health care answered by scientific research. The abortion debate as an issue for ethical enquiry necessitates some knowledge of ethical theory and basic ethical principles to develop an understanding of the moral issues involved. Philosophical ethical theories provide a framework that underpins an ethical outlook (Benjamin and Curtis, 1992), and there are many ethical theories along a continuum that stretches from utilitarianism to deontology. Discussion of the two main traditional schools, utilitarianism and deontology, aids in the comprehension of the principles behind the framework. Utilitarianism is the prevailing goal-based theory associated with the goal of happiness or pleasure, and the concept of 'the greatest good for the greatest number' (Seedhouse and Lovett, 1992). Jeremy Bentham (1748–1832) and John Stuart Mill (1806–1873) are famously associated with utilitarianism and the 'greatest happiness principle'. Deontology, or non-consequentialism, is a duty-based theory, placing duty above consequences. The moral philosophy of Immanual Kant (1724–1802) is influential in a deontological ethical framework, where the concept of duty is more important than the concept of maximizing good for the majority. For Kant, it is not the end result of an act that makes it right or wrong, but rather the moral intention of the agent (Thompson *et al.*,

1994). The fundamental difference between the theories is that the former looks ahead to the consequences of the actions, while the latter looks back to the nature of the action itself (Palmer, 1995). Moral reasoning that flows from these ethical theories can be applied to the abortion issue to understand the different and often opposing moral arguments involved. From a deontological perspective, rational beings must be treated as an end in themselves, and never merely as a means to an end. However, if a pregnancy were the result of rape, autonomy of the woman would be neglected if abortion were denied – she would be treated as a means towards an end in circumstances that are not the result of her autonomous decision. Thus, abortion is allowed in these particular circumstances (Singleton and McLaren, 1995). The consequentialist view of abortion generally supports the liberal view, and considers the consequences of performing or not performing the abortion, which allows for a shift in values (Fletcher *et al.*, 1995). For example, making abortion illegal would be to the detriment of society. Illegal abortions would still be carried out, probably increasing maternal deaths, which decreased dramatically following the 1967 Abortion Act (Mundy *et al.*, 1989). Rumbold (1986) argues that in the 1967 Abortion Act, the utilitarian principle of the greatest happiness for the greatest number applies.

Thiroux (1995) describes five interdependent principles to be applied to any situation, including abortion:

1. The value of life
2. Goodness or rightness
3. Justice or fairness
4. Truth-telling or honesty
5. Individual freedom.

The principle of 'the value of life' is seen as the first principle, because without it the others are meaningless (Burnard and Chapman, 1993). Tschudin (1992) contends 'the value of life' to be a near absolute principle, and if abortion is viewed in the context of killing it transgresses this principle. However, Thiroux (1995) asserts that quality as well as quantity of life has to be considered as an important aspect within the abortion debate, given the situation of an unwanted child or a child born with a serious genetic abnormality. The principle of individual freedom is also important in the abortion debate; the mother's right of self-determination is a central issue. The ANP must provide support so that an informed decision can be made.

This does not mean that the remaining three principles, goodness or rightness, justice or fairness, and truth-telling or honesty, are not applicable. Indeed, as Burnard and Chapman (1993) explain, if right and good are demonstrated by the individual's conscience, there is unresolvable conflict between a pro-life and pro-choice position; each will follow their own conscience. Individual freedom as a principle applied to abortion will be discussed with regard to freedom of the mother and freedom of the fetus. The above principles are seen as interdependent. As Tschudin (1992) clarifies, without freedom there is no morality; freedom is required to synthesize the other four ethical principles.

Another set of complementary ethical principles promoted by Gillon (1986) underpin practice and provide a framework for discussion of moral dilemmas, and thus may be applied to the abortion debate. These are autonomy, justice, beneficence and non-maleficence. Autonomy is the right to self-determination and personal freedom, and is therefore closely related to the concept of personhood, an issue that will shortly be discussed more fully in relation to the problem of when life begins. Respect for the autonomy of a pregnant women's decision to terminate her pregnancy is an obligation for health care professionals. Nevertheless, there are procedures in place to protect the personal autonomy of health care workers who disagree with abortion, in the form of conscientious objection (Dimond, 1999). Even so, the woman must be treated with respect, dignity and understanding at all times. The principles of beneficence and non-maleficence must be viewed with respect to patient autonomy in the practitioner's own decision-making process. For example, a doctor may perceive an abortion to be a great harm and something that should be avoided (non-maleficence). Alternatively, a pregnant teenager may consider proceeding with an unwanted pregnancy to be a greater long-term harm, and that termination of her pregnancy is something that she can cope with without too much physical and psychological trauma (beneficence).

The legal position

In acting as an advocate for the client who seeks a termination of pregnancy, the advanced practitioner must be aware of the laws concerning abortion. Abortion laws differ greatly throughout the world. Abortion is available on request up to 10–12 weeks' gestation in 13 European countries and at up to 12 weeks' gestation in some states in America, subject to legislative control (Davies, 1991). In the UK, abortion is not available on request. To have a legal abortion, the criteria of the 1967 Abortion Act, as amended in 1990 by The Human Fertilisation and Embryology Act, have to be fulfilled. This law does not apply to Northern Ireland and the Republic of Ireland. There is room for liberal interpretation of the law, although two medical practitioners must consent to the woman's request to terminate her pregnancy and agree that one of the five clauses are met. The majority of abortions are performed under clauses C and D of the Act, which are referred to in practice as 'social' reasons; that the continued pregnancy would threaten the woman's mental health or the health of her existing children. Clauses A, B and E are identified as medical reasons for abortion, clause E relating to abnormalities of the fetus (Paterson, 1998).

The role of the medical profession as 'gatekeepers' in obtaining abortion has resulted from the power vested in doctors in shaping the 1960s abortion laws (Peterson, 1993). Furthermore, from a historical perspective the medicalization of the reproductive health of women has resulted in medical paternalism, undermining the rights of women and the value of self-determination. In Sweden there is little public controversy over the abortion issue. First trimester abortions are available on request and all members of the health care team are involved, each contributing with their own area of expertise and providing the care and support that values the woman's autonomy (Peterson, 1993).

The abortion issue in the USA is a bitterly fought battle, with diversity of opinion stretching over a seemingly irreducible chasm. Dworkin (1993) argues that conflict in the USA is partly due to the way the law was created, through the sole fiat of the Supreme Court. Interestingly, the concept of advanced practice evolved from the USA. Expansion of roles in the British health care system, as in the USA, is expected to provide benefits dictated by the current economic and social climate (Dunn, 1997). While practitioners in the USA do not have a legal or moral duty to take part in abortion care, they do have a duty to treat any patient with dignity, respect and understanding (Curtin, 1993). Widespread and strong religious convictions and opposing opinions from a strong feminist movement also fuel the controversy in the USA.

Religious and cultural issues

Religious traditions and cultural diversity are inextricably linked to the abortion issue and many other ethical dilemmas. Religion, it may be claimed, forms the basis of ethics and moral reasoning. However, as Benjamin and Curtis (1992) argue, this is a fallacious assumption; secular considerations also support basic ethical principles in pluralistic society and prevent absolutism. The ancient Christians distinguished between the unquickened fetus and the quickened fetus, when fetal movements were perceived, and abortion then became a sin or a crime (Peterson, 1993). In Great Britain, abortions before quickening were not considered to be a crime before 1803. The timing of ensoulment (entry into the embryo of the spiritual soul) has changed throughout history, yet until 1869, when the absolutist position was established, Roman Catholicism accepted the view that only destruction of the fetus following ensoulment at quickening was considered a serious crime (Kenyon, 1986). Protestantism has varying views on abortion and, unlike the Roman Catholic religion, sexuality does not play a crucial role. Sociologist Kristin Luker, cited by Steinbock (1992), argues that differing views on the meaning and value of sexuality and the roles of women are factors that influence views on abortion and the status of the fetus. In reality, fundamentalism is not widespread; in our modern society, with religious authority diminishing, Roman Catholic views on abortion range from strongly pro-life to more moderate positions.

The abortion argument

Opinions on abortion are often categorized, although there may be differences of opinion within each category. Anti-abortion, pro-life or conservative groups all maintain that abortion is wrong. Their argument is based on the principle of the value or sanctity of life and the genetic view of the beginning of human life whereby a human being emerges at conception, and it is wrong to kill an innocent human being. Arguments against abortion also include the domino argument (Thiroux, 1995). This argument, it is claimed, is exemplified by the Nazi atrocities, which began with the legalization of abortion. This results in disregard for innocent human life and leads to complete disregard for all human life. Anti-abortion arguments may also include (Thiroux, 1995):

- The medical and psychological dangers to pregnant women
- The need to consider alternative options such as adoption
- Acceptance and responsibility if pregnancy is the result of a sexual relationship
- If the pregnancy is a result of rape or incest, that the fetus is the innocent victim.

Liberal views, pro-choice arguments for abortion, argue that the decision should be undertaken by the pregnant woman, who is in the best position to make that decision, thus upholding the principle of individual freedom. The moral status of the fetus may be rejected or even accepted to a degree; nonetheless, consideration of the fetus is subordinate to that of the mother (Fletcher *et al.*, 1995). This may also be considered to be a deontological view. Extreme liberals accept abortion on demand at any stage of pregnancy, but most pro-choice views take fetal development into consideration. Late abortions have greater potential risks for the women, both physically and psychologically, but should not be denied, for example, in the case of fetal abnormality. Counter-arguments to the pro-life view refute the domino argument, which lacks evidence to show that legal abortion will disrespect other areas of human life (Thiroux, 1995). Abortion is also a relatively safe medical procedure. It is illegal abortions that are generally unsafe, and these would be the consequence if laws on abortion were restricted. Thus, abortion should always be legal and allowed in order to protect the safety of those women who seek termination of their pregnancy.

Psychological sequelae

Research papers on the psychological sequelae of abortion agree that adverse reactions occur in only a minority of women (Gilchrist, 1998). Indeed, it may be argued that psychological damage would be greater if a woman were forced to care for an unwanted or deformed child (Thiroux, 1995). Alternatives to abortion, such as adoption, are considered poor options, and if women are responsible for their sexual activities then abortion is a necessary component in reproductive care. Rape and incest are vile crimes, and thus it is argued that there can be no justification to make a woman suffer the continuation of a pregnancy in these distressing circumstances. However, pro-life proponents would argue for the 'sanctity' of the innocent life. It may also be argued that the state has no business in establishing laws on abortion (Singer, 1993). While alternative moral convictions must be tolerated, the decision regarding abortion is very much the woman's choice, and laws must not impose on this right.

Feminist theories

In this exciting and challenging era in the development of the profession of nursing, feminist theories have become more influential. The role of the ANP is to provide a service that is equal to and complementary to medicine. The advanced practitioner will perform activities previously within the medical domain, focusing on a holistic, caring approach rather than simulating the curative medical model. As Booth *et al.* (1997) suggest, feminist approaches in nursing have resulted from challenging the gender bias in health care and the predominance of the 'medical model'. Feminist opinions on abortion may differ within the feminist movement, but are generally on the far liberal end of the spectrum. In her discussion on feminist and medical ethics, Sherwin (1992) argues that within medical ethics the abortion debate is focused on philosophical arguments, isolating abortion decisions from other aspects of women's lives. Feminist medical ethics seeks to include the abortion decision as reproductive choice and reproductive freedom without neglecting and addressing other inequalities inherent in our patriarchal society. Gilligan, in her famous research on the moral dilemma of abortion (cited by Larrabee, 1993), argues that women think about moral decisions in a different way to men, paying more attention to the ethic of care. The women in the study were undoubtedly troubled by the decision they faced, yet the uncertainty was not related to philosophical arguments on the personhood of the fetus with a right to life; rather, they concentrated on the implications associated with their everyday life. Gilligan's work has been criticized, particularly her methodology (Larrabee, 1993), but the value of her work is important in recognizing the holistic character of moral problems and how they relate to everyday life rather than relying solely on the abstract concepts of ethicists. In another frequently cited study a feminist argument is presented by the philosopher Judith Thomson (Palmer, 1995). Thomson's analogy with the famous violinist is designed to focus on the property rights of women (Sherwin, 1992). Thomson accepts that fetal human development is continuous and personhood granted at any time is an arbitrary decision. She argues that fetal right to life is subordinate to the women's right to self-defence when the pregnancy is due to rape or the mother's life is threatened, and the ownership rights of her own body to expel an unwanted foreign body. When applied to Thomson's analogy, from a utilitarian stance it would be wrong to disconnect from the violinist as greater good may be achieved by him remaining attached. Although, through the popularity of self-interest, disconnection may prove to be a popular choice and would not be totally rejected given the sacrifice involved (Singer, 1993). In opposition to Thomson's view, Brody (in Bandman and Bandman, 1995) argues that the moral status of the fetus and the mother are equal and therefore they have the same right to life, so abortion is not morally permissible.

Conflicts of rights

Conflicts of rights between the mother and the fetus are a fundamental issue in the abortion debate. Rights, both moral and legal, are justified claims which impose on others to act in a certain way or refrain from acting in a certain way, thus imposing positive and/or negative duties on others (Thompson *et al.*, 1994). In English law a woman does not have a right to abortion; doctors control that right. Similarly, the father of the fetus has no rights in a decision to terminate a pregnancy; this is often challenged in legal arguments and consequently dismissed (Harris, 1991). The father cannot impose duties on the mother, for to force a woman to continue an unwanted pregnancy would constitute a grave physical assault upon her (Harris, 1991). Nor does the fetus have legal rights. In common law the fetus has no civil personality; rights are established at birth when personhood is established in law (Beazley, 1994). Warren (1992) argues that to extend legal rights to the fetus threatens a woman's right to choose abortion. It is not possible to give equal rights to the fetus, when the fetus is inside the woman, without encroachment on her basic rights. Warren, like Tooley (1983), is a proponent of the 'person view' (Steinbock, 1992). In this view a human fetus is genetically human; however, it is only persons rather than genetic humans who have a right to life. A descriptive 'person's' right to life is based on the 'interest' principle; for Tooley, only beings that have interests have rights. Critics of this view point out a new born infant also has no interests and thus has no strong right to life, a view they find morally repugnant. Tooley (1983) actually claims late abortion and early infanticide are not an intrinsic moral wrong. Warren (1992) is not as definite in her views on infanticide and late abortion; she accepts late gestation fetuses have substantial moral standing, although the autonomy of the mother should never be overridden. Warren's support for abortion, like Steinbock's (1992), is not solely based on a woman's right to choose what happens to her body, as this produces a narrow argument. Neither should support be solely based on the premise that the fetus lacks moral status, as potentiality arguments come into force whereby the fetus has the potential to obtain characteristics of personhood, therefore it may be accorded something like full moral status and hence abortion should not be performed. Rather, the argument is augmented by combining both approaches. McLachlan (1997) argues that pro-choice arguments based on the right to bodily self-determination are flawed – entitlement to abortion cannot be assumed from a moral entitlement to do what we want with our bodies, since there is no such entitlement. Interestingly, the sanctity of life argument influenced by Catholicism rests on the fetus's right to life. An abortion is, in strict interpretation, a wrong only allowed to God, who has a monopoly on rights (Botros, 1994).

Philosophical views

Philosophical views about abortion include the concept of personhood and the problems of when life begins and when life matters morally. The ways in which we think about this concept, the personhood or non-personhood of the fetus, has implications for the debate about abortion. When does personhood or self begin? For Grobstein (cited by Harris, 1991), self is personhood, which makes us 'characteristically different'. Warren (1972, in Tschudin, 1994, p. 37) offers five criteria to be fulfilled to become a person: consciousness; reasoning; self-motivated activity; the capacity to communicate, and the presence of self-concepts and self-awareness. Moderate views on abortion dispute the strong pro-life view that personhood dates from conception; it is only later in gestation that the fetus may fulfil some of Waren's criteria. Like Tooley (1983), Singer (1993) takes the argument a step further when he argues that a newborn infant is not a rational self-conscious being and so, like the fetus, has no claim to life as a person. The moderate or 'interest' view (Steinbock, 1992) states that embryos and early fetuses lack moral status and do not have interests, so personhood is not attained until some later point in development, like sentience and/or viability. This developmental viewpoint considers that human rights develop as biological life develops. When the fetus has sufficient value, it has accumulated the same rights as a newborn infant. For Singer (1993), given its lack of self-awareness etc., the fetus does not have the same claim to life. Indeed, Singer argues that pro-lifers are biased *Homo sapiens* if they eat animals killed at a far more advanced level than that of the fetus (Singer, 1993).

The value of fetal life, and the need for ethics to be responsive, is central to the debate. Disagreement on abortion actually stems from the interpretation of sanctity. 'Detached objection' to abortion is concerned with the sanctity of human life (Dworkin, 1993), and this view does not suggest that the fetus has interests. The 'derivative objection' to abortion assigns rights and interests to the fetus equal to those of all members of the moral community. The question of whether the fetus is a person is filled with ambiguities and is therefore unhelpful. The sacredness of life is valued by all; what differs is the interpretation and complexities of these values.

As a non-sentient being the fetus has no moral rights – even towards full term the fetus fulfils fewer criteria for personhood than an adult fish (Steinbock, 1992). As fetal development continues, the point at which sentience occurs and the situation changes is debatable (Campbell *et al.*, 1997). Singer (1993) argues that when the fetus is conscious and can feel pain abortion is an extremely difficult decision (as it is at any stage), but the woman's interests still override those of a sentient fetus (Singer, 1993).

Potentiality arguments in the purist form insist that from conception the potential for a new human being is present, and it should therefore be treated as an actual human being. Counter-arguments to this claim are often discussed in terms of contraception or the analogy of the development of an acorn to an oak. Contraception is accepted by most people, and, according to the potentiality argument, the ovum and the sperm as potential life means that abortion and contraception are morally equal (Tooley, 1983). Medico-legal opinion agrees that contraceptive methods that work before implantation are not abortive (French, 1998). The view that viability and sentience mark a point at which abortion is unacceptable is open to criticism. Viability relies a great deal on medical technology, which differs throughout the world. Today a fetus of 22 weeks' gestation has a slim chance of survival, but 20 years ago this would not have been possible (Ballantyne, 1998). Abortion laws generally rely on viability criteria, with fetal protection after viability replacing the woman's right to self-determination (Steinbock, 1992). Sentience may mark a morally significant point; however, the onset of sentience is not an exact science, although recently scientific evidence of sentient behaviour is placed at 26 weeks' gestation (Royal College of Obstetricians and Gynaecologists (RCOG) 1997). 'Brain birth' may also be chosen as a suitable point to mark fetal protection, and is placed at 20 weeks' gestation to account for errors in gestational age. Steinbock (1992) believes that sentience is preferable to 'brain birth', as it marks a qualitative difference in the life of the unborn.

Potentiality arguments may have different and extreme interpretations. As a moderate argument with a gradualist emphasis it is a popular ethical stance and contributes to moral reasoning in the abortion debate. Scientists, ethicists, geneticists and theologians will continue to debate when a fetus should be regarded as a person. The practitioner providing reproductive sexual health services requires an ethical understanding on the abortion issue in order to assist the woman and/or couple to make an informed choice.

The role of the advanced nurse practitioner

Expansion in the role of practice nurses, particularly in providing sexual health services, looks set to continue as primary care seeks to function more efficiently (Madden, 2000). According to the RCOG (2000), at least one-third of women experience an abortion before the age of 45 years. Research for Schering Health Care (Family Planning Association, 1996) showed that nationwide over 850 000 women were at risk of an unintended pregnancy. These statistics, together with new abortion guidelines by the RCOG and expansion in the role of the practice nurse, mean that nurses in primary care will be involved with unintended pregnancies in their day-to-day practice. Germaine Greer (2000) argues that not before time has the RCOG recognized that inconsistencies and delay in the provision of abortion will not be tolerated. As a consequence of the White Paper on the NHS (Department of Health, 1997) the concept of clinical governance was introduced to set standards of quality throughout the NHS spectrum of care. Dimond (1999) advised clarification and nationwide uniformity of standards for women requesting abortion, and the new abortion guidelines appear to have responded to Dimond's request. Confirmation of inequitable access and variation in the quality of abortion care was provided by a national audit when the new guidelines were launched (*Practice Nursing News*, 2000). Following the philosophy of clinical governance, the guidelines aim to set standards of good practice to be incorporated in the production of local protocols.

The UK has the highest teenage conception rate in Western Europe; before the age of 20, one in eight women in Britain has a child (Health Education Authority, 1999). Governmental priority to reduce teenage conception rates has implications to improve sexual health provision to young people in primary care. The provision of sexual health services by practice nurses was investigated by Stokes and Mears (2000), whose research concluded there was scope to improve the provision in general practice, particularly in relation to services to teenagers. Unwanted teenage pregnancies can have catastrophic effects on the young person involved in both social and economic terms. According to research, GP practices with a younger female GP had fewer teenage pregnancies (Hippisley-Cox *et al.*, 2000). The research concluded that there may be scope for developing sexual health service to teenagers by practice nurses, the majority of whom are female. Moreover, Wooton (1995) found that nurses were perceived as being more approachable than doctors.

Many nurses working in general practice have relinquished their traditional roles to perform activities previously felt to be within the doctor's remit. Rather than following a medical curative model, many nurses follow the philosophy of 'human existentialism'. The client then emerges as the central focus, making informed choices through holistic care that will ultimately lead to empowerment, one of the goals of the advanced practitioner role. The role of the ANP is multifaceted, and definitions of advanced practice accordingly lack conceptual clarity; analysis of the role is not an easy task. However, recent NHS guidance on the role of the advanced practitioner attempts to clarify matters. *Making a Difference* (DoH, 1999) renames ANPs as 'nurse consultants'. Core skills and competencies of the nurse consultant post will be devised in conjunction with the UKCC's recommendations for a higher level of practice (UKCC, 1999). Whilst educational, training and clinical responsibilities have become clearer, the nurse consultant, like the ANP, will provide high quality care with a high degree of professional autonomy (Castledine, 1999). It may be envisaged this degree of professional autonomy will assist in reaching the goals in abortion practice.

The impact of recent reforms in the community context are immense, and doubtless these reforms will continue at an unrelenting pace into the new century. Whilst there are problems with advancing nursing practice, not least in the lack of clarity of role definition, the ANP is in a unique position to deliver high quality sexual health care. The different way in which ANPs can communicate with clients requesting abortion will facilitate a major responsibility of advanced practitioners – that is, to empower their clients (Snyder and Mirr, 1995). The ethical dimension to the abortion debate requires careful consideration as the ANP makes professional autonomous decisions and seeks to empower the client. Empowerment changes the knowledge base (Rodwell, 1996) and, through education, patients can increase their control over their lives and health, shifting the power base.

The advanced practitioner may see clients with an unintended pregnancy in a family planning clinic or during general surgery time. The specialist knowledge and highly developed skills the ANP has acquired are invaluable in receiving this client. If the client then requests an abortion, the ANP cannot sign to say the client has met any of the criteria of the Abortion Act. However, depending on local policy, the ANP could then refer without delay to a specialist organization, such as the British Pregnancy Advisory Service, where two medical practitioners may sign the relevant legal documents. The therapeutic relationship the ANP develops with the client during the initial consultation is invaluable in providing continuity of care. Following the abortion procedure the client may return at any stage for whatever reason directly to the ANP, assisting in the provision of a seamless high quality service.

Summary

The abortion debate has many components and relates to many other ethical dilemmas – for example, embryo experimentation and euthanasia. This chapter has discussed a range of views and accepts the right of individuals to hold those views. However, there are strong arguments for leaving the decision to the person who is in the best position to make that decision – the pregnant woman – whilst still accepting the right of conscientious objection by some health care workers and the fact that certain gestational time limits are valid. Safe, early abortion with equality of provision for this service is a necessary part of reproductive health care. The decision to terminate a pregnancy may involve ethical considerations that are equally applicable to other ethical decisions, and may also involve reasons that are unique to the woman; thus it cannot be viewed in an abstract way. Late abortions, which raise the strongest objections, are relatively rare, and energy should be channelled into offering an improved service to reduce all unwanted pregnancies. Members of the primary health care team, especially ANPs, are in a prime position to offer support and non-judgemental advice to women making decisions about abortion and many other ethical dilemmas. The ethical issues involved in the abortion debate require ethical knowledge, which will lead to greater ethical understanding and moral reasoning and ultimately to an improved holistic service for all clients.

Key points

- Abortion is a highly emotive, divisive and complex issue.
- Abortion will continue to be a necessary component in women's reproductive health care.
- Philosophical views on abortion are discussed in terms of personhood and the complex issues of when life begins and when life matters morally.
- The debate reveals the conflict and complexities between 'pro-choice' and 'pro-life' groups, and the principles of individual freedom and of the value or sanctity of life.
- New abortion guidelines seek to provide safe, early abortion, with equality of access to abortion services.
- The autonomous role of the ANP seeking to empower clients through an holistic nursing service will assist in the provision of high quality sexual health care.
- ANPs require a deep understanding of ethical dilemmas to increase their capacity for advanced clinical reasoning, which is a necessary competency of their role.

References

Adams, A., Pelletier, D., Duffield, C. *et al.* (1997). Determining and discerning expert practice: a review of the literature. *Clin. Nurse Spec.*, **11(5)**, 217–21.

Autar, R. (1996). The *Scope of Professional Practice* in specialist practice. *Br. J. Nursing*, **5(16)**, 984–90.

Ballantyne, A. (1998). Born survivors. *The Times Magazine*, 21 March.

Bandman, E. and Bandman, B. (1995). *Nursing Ethics Through the Life Span.* Prentice Hall.

Beazley, J. (1994). Does a fetus have rights? In: *Ethics in Obstetrics and Gynaecology* (S. Bewley and H. Ward, eds), pp. 81–9. RCOG.

Benjamin, M. and Curtis, J. (1992). *Ethics in Nursing*. Oxford University Press.

BMA (1998). *Medical Ethics Today: Its Practice and Philosophy*. BMJ Publishing Group.

Booth, K., Kenrick, M and Woods, S. (1997). Nursing knowledge, theory and method revisited. *J. Adv. Nursing*, **26**, 804–11.

Botros, S. (1994). What's wrong with rights? In: *Ethics in Obstetrics and Gynaecology* (S. Bewley and H. Ward, eds), pp. 90–7. RCOG.

Burnard, P. and Chapman, C. M. (1993). *Professional and Ethical Issues in Nursing*. Scutari Press.

Campbell, A., Charlesworth, M., Gillett, G and Jones, G. (1997). *Medical Ethics*. Oxford University Press.

Castledine, G. (1999). Nurse consultants herald a new era for clinical nursing. *Br. J. Nursing*, **5(8)**, 1258.

Clarke, L. (1999). The person in abortion. *Nursing Ethics*, **6(1)**, 37–44.

Curtin, L. (1993). Abortion: a tangle of rights. *Nursing Management*, **24 Jan**, 26–30.

Davies, V. (1991). *Abortion and Afterwards*. Ashgrove Press Limited.

Department of Health (1997) *The New NHS: Modern and Dependable*. HMSO.

Department of Health (1999) *Making a Difference: Strengthening the Nursing, Midwifery and Health Visiting Contribution to Health and Health Care*. DoH.

Dimond, B. (1999). A legal right to abortion: right or wrong?. *Br. J. Midwifery*, **7(6)**, 355–7.

Dunn, L. (1997). A literature review of advanced clinical nursing practice in the United States of America. *J. Adv. Nursing*, **25**, 814–19.

Dworkin, R. (1993). *Life's Dominion*. Harper Collins.

Dyson, L. and White, A. (1999). Termination of pregnancy: a difficult decision-making process. *Br. J. Community Nursing*, **4(9)**, 476–82.

Edwards, M. (1997). Patient autonomy. *Practice Nurse*, **14(3)**, 206–8.

Family Planning Association (1996). *Contraceptive Education Bulletin*. FPA.

Fletcher, N., Holt, J., Brazier, M. and Harris, J. (eds). (1995). *Ethics Law and Nursing*. Manchester University Press.

French, K. (1998). Family planning – a moral dilemma? *Practice Nurse*, **15(10)**, 587–9.

Fryer, N. (1995). How useful is a knowledge of ethics? *Br. J. Midwifery*, **3(6)**, 343–5.

Gilchrist, A. C. (1998). Psychological sequelae of abortion. *Trends Urol. Gynaecol. Sexual Health*, **March**.

Gillon, R. (1986). *Philosophical Medical Ethics*. John Wiley and Sons.

Greer, G. (2000). Abortion policy finally catches up with reality. *Nursing Times*, **96(13)**, 8.

Harris, J. (1991). *The Value of Life*. Routledge.

Health Education Authority (1999). *Reducing the Rate of Teenage Conceptions. An International Review of the Evidence from Europe*. Summary bulletin, Health Education Authority.

Hippisley-Cox, J., Allen, J., Pringle, M., Edbon, D., McPhearson, M., Churchill, D. and Bradley, S. (2000). Association between teenage pregnancy rates and the age and sex of GPs: cross sectional survey in Trent 1994–97. *Br. Med. J.*, **320**, 842–5.

Kenyon, E. (1986). *The Dilemma of Abortion.* Faber and Faber.

Larrabee, M. J. (ed.). (1993). *An Ethic of Care.* Routledge.

Loudon, N., Glassier, A. and Gebbie, A. (1995). *Handbook of Family Planning and Reproductive Care.* Churchill Livingstone.

Madden, V. (2000). Health experts advocate the expanded role of the nurse. *Practice Nurse*, **19(5)**, 193.

Malik, M. (1997). Advocacy in nursing – a review of the literature. *J. Adv. Nursing*, **25**, 130–38.

McLachlan, H. V. (1997). Bodies, rights and abortion. *J. Med. Ethics*, **23**, 176–80.

Mundy, D., Francome, C. and Savage, W. (1989). Twenty-one years of legal abortion. *Br. Med. J.*, **298**, 1231–4.

Office for National Statistics (2000). *Abortion Statistics 1998.* The Stationery Office.

Palmer, M. (1995) *Moral Problems.* The Lutterworth Press.

Paterson, C. (1998). Induced abortion, part 1. *Trends Urol. Gynaecol. Sexual Health*, **March**.

Peterson, K. A. (1993). *Abortion Regimes.* Dartmouth.

Practice Nursing News (2000). New abortion guidelines. *Practice Nursing*, **11**, 12.

Rodwell, C. M. (1996). An analysis of the concept of empowerment. *J. Adv. Nursing*, **23**, 305–13.

Royal College of Obstetricians and Gynaecologists (1997). Summary and recommendations. In: *Fetal Awareness. Report of a Working Party.* ROCG.

Royal College of Obstetricians and Gynaecologists (2000). *Evidence-based Guideline on the Care of Women Requesting Abortion.* ROCG.

Rumbold, G. (1986). *Ethics in Nursing Practice.* Bailliere Tindall.

Seedhouse, D. and Lovett, L. (1992). *Practical Medical Ethics.* John Wiley and Sons.

Sherwin, S. (1992). Feminist and medical ethics: two different approaches to contextual ethics. In: *Feminist Perspectives in Medical Ethics* (H. Bequaert Holmes and L. M. Purdy, eds), pp. 17–31. Indiana University Press.

Singer, P. (1993). *Practical Ethics.* Cambridge University Press.

Singleton, J. and McLaren, S. (1995). *Ethical Foundations of Health Care.* Mosby.

Snyder, M. and Mirr, M. (eds). (1995). *Advanced Nursing Practice.* Springer.

Steinbock, B. (1992). *Life Before Birth.* Oxford University Press.

Stokes, T. and Mears, J. (2000). Sexual health and the practice nurse: a survey of reported practice attitudes. *Br. J. Family Planning*, **26(2)**, 89–92.

Thiroux, J. P. (1995). *Ethics: Theory and Practice.* Prentice Hall.

Thompson, I. E., Melia, K. M. and Boyd, K. M. (1994). *Nursing Ethics.* Churchill Livingstone.

Tooley, M. (1983). *Abortion and Infanticide.* Clarendon Press.

Tschudin, V. (1992). *Ethics in Nursing.* Butterworth-Heinemann.

Tschudin, V. (1994). *Deciding Ethically.* Bailliere Tindall.
United Kingdom Central Council (1992). *The Scope of Professional Practice.* UKCC.
United Kingdom Central Council (1999). *A Higher Level of Practice.* UKCC.
Warren, M. A. (1992). The moral significance of birth. In: *Feminist Perspectives in Medical Ethics* (H. Bequaert Holmes and L. M. Purdy, eds), pp. 32–45. Indiana University Press.
Wooton, G. (1995), *The Nurse's Role in the Provision of Emergency Contraception.* RCOG, Faculty of Family Planning and Reproductive Care.

Raising awareness of the ethical issues surrounding termination of pregnancy for fetal abnormalities

Pamela Campbell

Introduction

Advanced nurse practitioners (ANPs) working within primary care or midwifery are likely at some point in their career to encounter the emotive experience of supporting women whose unborn child is found to be abnormal. The care and support needed for these women, who may opt for termination or continuation of the pregnancy, is considerable and far-reaching. ANPs, with their unique blend of knowledge, sensitivity and excellent communication skills, are therefore ideal professionals to provide optimum care. However, this means that ANPs need to have thought through the ethical issues linked with abortion for fetal abnormality. This chapter thus sets out many of the ethical areas that need to be considered when supporting women in this traumatic situation. It is hoped that by raising awareness of these issues, ANPs may be better prepared to aid women with their acute and distressing decision-making process.

The ethical dilemma of deciding to continue with a pregnancy or to terminate the life of a blighted fetus is one that could potentially arise for any pregnant woman. Almost every woman embarking on a pregnancy from choice does so with the anticipation of achieving a full-term, healthy, normal infant. However, it is estimated that 2 per cent of pregnancies will result in some form of abnormality. Kenyon (1986) reports that around 14 000 babies are born in the UK each year with some form of congenital defect. The rapidly advancing technology of molecular genetics and the development of prenatal screening techniques have ensured that induced abortion for fetal abnormalities remains a topic in need of rigorous moral analysis. The question of whether abortion is morally justifiable has raged throughout the ages.

Anthropological studies reveal that abortion has been widely practised across cultures and throughout history (Johnstone, 1994). Prenatal screening, which emerged in the twentieth century, added another moral dimension to the age-old debate, and the discovery of the complete genetic code in the new millennium has sharpened the ethical debate still further.

Before moving on to discuss issues surrounding abortion, it is important to clarify the terminology used. This helps to avoid the potential for emotive bias that may occur from misunderstanding of the term 'abortion'. A dictionary definition of 'the expulsion of the fetus from the uterus before the age of viability' will be adopted herein. Abortion may be spontaneous (commonly termed as miscarriage), or induced for therapeutic reasons. Induced abortion, also referred to as termination of pregnancy, is the subject of focus in this chapter. The Abortion Act of 1967 legalized therapeutic abortion, and an amendment by the Human Fertilisation and Embryology Act in 1990 specified that in the event of severe fetal abnormality abortion may be legally performed at any stage of pregnancy in order to prevent suffering to the mother and child.

Looking back 20–30 years (or more), it appeared to be an accepted fact that some mothers would give birth to babies with severe abnormalities. Such tragedies were seen as inevitable and unavoidable; they were accepted as an 'Act of God', an unfortunate occurrence outside human control. Today technological advances in prenatal screening have changed the situation. Most abnormalities can now be detected antenatally through blood tests, analysis of amniotic fluid, or ultrasound scanning. Parents attending for screening will be made aware if the fetus is abnormal, and given the choice whether to continue the pregnancy or to terminate the life of the fetus before it is born in order to avoid a lifetime of disability. An ethical dilemma has thus been created by technological advances in obstetric screening.

ANPs involved in the care of these women require the ability to review the ethical crisis objectively and comprehensively. Their resultant clarity of views will expose appropriate routes whereby they are able to guide women through the moral maze of abortion. With a heightened awareness of issues involved, it may be that ANPs can reduce the emotional battering of their patients in this situation by anticipating and understanding some possible views that may be expressed within the decision-making process.

When does life begin?

Attitudes towards abortion are often determined by an individual's views on when life begins. The dating of pregnancy is determined by the first day of the last menstrual period – i.e. this is theoretically classed as day one of pregnancy, whereas in reality this is prior to conception. Pro-life supporters see the beginning of life as the formation of the zygote – that is, the group of cells resulting from the union of the ovum and sperm. Supporters of this view include the Roman Catholic Church, and their views logically extend to condemn the use of those contraceptives that achieve their function following a fusion of sperm and egg (e.g. intrauterine devices) as well as all abortions.

Less radical views see the embryo as the start of life, which refers to the conceptus between the second and eighth weeks of gestation. Moderates refer to the beginning of life within the continuum of fetal development, which relates to the period from the eighth week of gestation to full-term. A fetus is fully formed from 12 weeks onwards, in the sense that all major organs are present although not mature.

Historically, the occurrence of 'quickening' (when the first fetal movements are felt by the mother) was often perceived as the beginning of life. However, it is now well established that the fetus is capable of movement long before this is actually felt by the mother, so the landmark of 'quickening' has become less significant. It is also pertinent to note that quickening usually occurs at an earlier stage of pregnancy in multiparous women. If quickening previously represented the earliest time that the mother was able to appreciate the fetus as a living entity, then this has also altered. Earlier antenatal bookings now mean that most women will have an ultrasound scan within the first trimester, at which time they will be able to see the fetal heart beating, and routine use of the Doppler at 12–14 weeks' gestation provides auditory evidence of the baby's existence. As a consequence, the mother may experience her unborn child as a tangible being at an earlier stage of pregnancy as a direct result of medical technology.

The fetal age of viability in the United Kingdom has been legally determined as 24 weeks' gestation (Human Fertilisation and Embryology Act, 1990). However, it is not correspondingly possible to determine a gestational age for personhood. The issue of personhood is central to the question of whether abortion is or is not morally permissible. Once it is recognized that a being is a person, it is also recognized that the being acquires moral rights (Warren, 1973).

When does personhood begin?

The question of when personhood develops is again one that can only be answered according to opinion rather than fact. Noonan (1970) states that the only non-arbitrary cut-off point between personhood and non-personhood is conception. The definition of personhood is in itself a complex matter, and without a clear definition the onset of personhood cannot be debated. Wells (1989) describes personhood concisely as 'an awareness of self as a present and future being'. Others see personhood as occurring once a brain is functioning. Brody (1975) sets this time as being between the sixth and twelfth weeks after conception, and therefore argues that abortion is acceptable up to this point. More precise definitions have been given by Tooley (1983) and Warren (1977), who stipulate that several demanding criteria must be met, including the capacity to arrive at decisions by deliberation. Tooley therefore takes the view that personhood can only be said to occur when a baby is aged 3 months, attributing this to physiological changes in the developing cortex that take 3 months to occur after birth. This is an extreme view and may logically extend to claim that infanticide is not wrong because it does not involve the killing of a 'person'. This is certainly an argument that ANPs should be aware of, but obviously consider within the context of legal boundaries.

If personhood is accepted as occurring only after birth then abortion should be free from moral questioning, as a fetus is not viewed as a person and therefore has no right to life. Harris (1985) supports the view that a fetus is not a person and therefore cannot be harmed if its life is ended prematurely. However, Harris also states that the fetus can be wronged in other ways – for example, by subjecting it to any pain – and therefore sees it as very important to ensure that abortion is made a painless process for the fetus. This seems a confused picture, where Harris is able to justify killing but not hurting a fetus. If a being is recognized as able to perceive pain, then this in itself may constitute a definition of personhood as it demonstrates both life and cognition. ANPs need to recognize that parents holding this view will need detailed explanation and reassurance about the practical procedures involved in the termination of pregnancy. Rational discussion regarding the death of the fetus prior to planned induction of labour may aid patients' decision making and possibly help to ease subsequent grief.

Other liberalists with an extreme view of personhood include Judith Jarvis Thomson (1971). She also argues that a fetus is not a person, and is in fact nothing more than a newly implanted clump of cells. However, she denies the relevance of the issue of personhood relating to abortion. Thomson argues that the only criterion as to whether abortion is permissible relates to the fact that a mother is not morally obliged to continue with a pregnancy if she did not wish the pregnancy to occur anyway. ANPs may need to remind antenatal women who are ridden with guilt at the thought of a termination that their own rights are also valid. ANPs must recognize that, when under pressure, women may give in to all sorts of demands or accommodate the needs of others rather than putting their own needs as a priority. This may lead to further discussion on assertiveness and honesty. By uncovering these areas ANPs may help patients to expose their true feelings, and thus empower them to make a decision that has hitherto been heavily influenced by others.

The ANP may also encounter the issue of personhood viewed in terms of potential personhood. This is where the emphasis is placed on the capacity of the fetus to develop into a potential person. The fundamentalist thus believes that the same right of life should apply to a potential life as to an actual life. This is a 'slippery slope' argument that can be tracked back to extremist views. If a fetus is a potential person, then so is an embryo, a zygote, an ovum, a sperm. Followers of this philosophy would therefore argue against contraception and ultimately also against celibacy. Glover (1977) claims that the issue of potential personhood places value on the potential rather than the actual fetus, and therefore justifies its termination.

However, referring to a fetus as a potential person is incorrect according to many. Fitzpatrick (1988) states that the notion of potentiality is confused with that of immaturity. This view maintains that all the characteristics for development into a person are actually present at conception, and therefore the conceptus is actually an immature person rather than a potential person. It is interesting to note that a person's level of maturity ordinarily has no bearing on the respect afforded to them. Fitzpatrick cites as an example that it is no worse a crime to kill a 16-year-old than a 6-year-old. This view therefore has a fundamental opposition to abortion, believing that it is unacceptable to use the immaturity of the fetus as an excuse for ending its life.

Parents who have previously espoused this view may need the ANP to remind them that this is just one way of interpreting personhood. This does not mean that the ANP is attempting to dissuade them from their beliefs, but rather recognizes that parents need to be fully informed prior to any decision-making. Part of the role of the ANP in this situation is to bring other perceptions into focus in order to clarify the wider picture. Conversely, this does not mean that the ANP will be exposing bewildered parents to a frightening moral melee they have never before recognized. The ANP will listen and respond to the parents' thoughts and help to expand them proportionately. Indeed, this is one reason why it requires a particularly skilled practitioner to support parents in this dilemma. Inexperienced nurses with little knowledge would fail to recognize the many complex issues that may need to be addressed, and nurses with a good knowledge but lacking in the delicate nuances that are so characteristic of the ANP may bewilder parents with an overwhelming array of ethical issues that they never wanted to consider.

The moral position of the fetus

The moderate's view on abortion perceives the fetus not as a human being, nor as a maternal appendage. The moral position of a fetus is recognized as unique, just as animals are recognized as having a unique status.

Moderates such as Wertheimer (1971) therefore argue that the fetus cannot be treated dishonourably because it is not merely an object, but neither does it need to be treated as a person because it is not a person. Abortion may therefore be viewed as being justifiable for the benefit of the fetus itself. If this stance is adopted a paternalistic approach is taken, whereby an assumption is made that it is preferable for the fetus to die rather than to live a life with disability. Is it possible to make this assumption? Many people with disabilities would strongly disagree.

The issue of rights is central to the abortion argument. Sutton (1990) identifies that some parents-to-be act as though they have a right to a healthy child, and feel that the medical profession is duty-bound to provide them with this. This is in fact an unreasonable request. Everything and everyone in life cannot be faultless, and this must be accepted as a natural fact. Followers of eugenics would not agree.

In legal terms, the position is simple. The fetus has no rights. The Congenital Disabilities (Civil Liability) Act, 1976 makes it impossible for a handicapped child to claim damages for 'wrongful life'. In lay terms, this means that a child (or adult) cannot sue for having been brought into existence as a result of negligent failure to act on a prenatal diagnosis of abnormality and procure an abortion. This is because of the impossible task of comparing the benefits of non-existence to life.

The law fails to recognize the rights of fathers to object to a partner's abortion, yet doctors have a recognized right to object to participate in abortion proceedings, as well as the right to form opinions in good faith as to whether abortion is justified. This puts the medical profession in a very paternalistic position. In legal terms it is not a woman's absolute right to have an abortion, although some argue that it should be (Thomson, 1971).

What does abnormality mean?

Permission for a woman to proceed with a termination must be granted by two doctors who are both in agreement. This means that doctors determine which conditions fall under the category of severe abnormality. It would be impossible to draw up a list with details of what constitutes severe abnormality that is acceptable to all.

People's views of what is abnormal inevitably vary. This is because the question of what is normal is also different for everyone. The ANP will need to raise individuals' awareness that their view of abnormality may be unique to them. Parents will need to recognize and trust their own views if they are to survive the hurt from criticism that may be directed at them by others with differing views. People are not clones. They are not identical. They all have imperfections and variations – this is part of being human. How is it thus possible to make a judgement on what is abnormal *in utero*? If normality equates to being intellectually intact, then any child suffering hypoxia at delivery may be seen as potentially intellectually impaired. Does this mean infanticide can be practised on these babies?

If abortion is justifiable on the grounds of fetal abnormality, then the distinction between what is normal and what is abnormal needs to be examined further. Just as the meaning of normal is different for everyone, similarly, the perception of degree of handicap is different for individuals. Experience of a particular handicap may determine individual attitudes towards this (Garrett and Carlton, 1994). For example, if a woman has a brother with Down's syndrome, she will have formed an opinion as to the quality of life experienced by people with Down's syndrome. This may be a negative or positive view, but will have been formed by personal experience rather than by purely objective consideration.

The concept of normality is also influenced by our own body image. The ANP must be particularly sensitive to this in cases where a pregnant woman has a congenital disability herself and finds that prenatal screening tests reveal that her fetus has the same condition. For example, a pregnant woman with achondroplasia may discover the child she is carrying also has achondroplasia. Would she consider this to be normal rather than abnormal? If the fetus did not have achondroplasia would she consider it abnormal, as it is different from her own body shape? Would she therefore be justified in seeking a termination of this pregnancy?

The question of what is normal may also be applied to racial factors. If a white woman is expecting a child fathered by a black man, would she consider the child to be abnormal because it had dark skin? If this could be demonstrated *in utero*, would she be justified in requesting an abortion because the child was abnormal in the sense that it had a different skin colour to her own?

These questions highlight the dilemma and arrogance of trying to determine what is and what is not normal. If the word 'different' was used instead of 'abnormal', this might make abortion difficult to justify in some cases. It is for this reason that ANPs need to be fully self-aware and inwardly to acknowledge any of their own prejudices.

Any discussion and attempts to define normality inevitably extend to adults who suffer from a disability. If abnormality is seen as sufficient grounds to justify killing any affected fetus, then this is the beginning of a 'slippery slope' argument that would justify the killing of a handicapped adult. The logical extension of the argument cannot be denied. Nazi Germany tried to argue this view, yet society rejected it as abhorrent. Some terminations may be performed for conditions such as spina bifida, yet this is a condition that many handicapped adults suffer from. This is undeniably sending a message of lack of value and degradation to those adults. Does it infer that the life of people with spina bifida is not worth living? Many people would be outraged by this suggestion.

The value of life

If society does not perceive handicapped adults to be less worthy than adults without disabilities, then it is not possible to say that deformed fetuses are any less valuable than perfect fetuses (Harris, 1985). Advocates of abortion because of fetal handicap are, however, saying that a potentially handicapped child is of less value than a normal child.

The comparative value of a normal versus handicapped life is another important angle to consider. Many people would say that they agreed with therapeutic termination of pregnancy if it was to prevent a lifetime of deformity and the inability to enjoy a full life. Yet who is able to judge what ' a life worth living' is?

The value of life principle has been summarized by Thiroux (1995) as 'Human beings should revere life and accept death'. He does not uphold the principle of 'life at all costs', but recognizes that no life can be everlasting. Thiroux would therefore not object to letting infants die if they had a condition that was incompatible with life, rather than artificially attempting to sustain life. Thiroux goes on to say that life is the one thing that all living human beings have in common, although each individual experiences life in a unique way – no one else can truly share or live another's life.

Yet the law dictates that the medical profession is placed in an arrogant position of determining whether a termination of pregnancy may be performed because abnormality would make that future child's life not worth living. If an assumption is made that people with abnormalities do have less worthwhile lives than others, it could be argued that it would be wrong for a woman not to have an abortion if she knew that she was carrying a severely abnormal child. This principle is supported by Glover (1976, p. 146), who states that:

> *The side effects of abortion will not in general be bad enough to outweigh the loss involved in bringing into the world someone whose life is much less worthwhile than that of a normal person who could be conceived instead.*

Glover also suggests that it is possible to replace one life (that of the abnormal fetus) with a subsequent healthy fetus. This is a further example of devaluing a life. Any mother who has lost a child and subsequently conceived another will testify that no life is replaceable. The ANP will have knowledge of bereavement processes and grief reactions, and will recognize that this attitude is artificial and could lead to problems in bonding with a subsequent child if the previous loss has not been fully accepted. Although it is only extremists who would concur with Glover's view, most moderates would agree that there is a point where life quality is so poor (as in PVS, persistent vegetative state) that the value of life is diminished. Rachels (1986, p. 5) believes that there:

> *. . . is a deep difference between having a life and merely being alive . . . Being alive in the biological' sense, is relatively unimportant. One's*

(biographical) life, by contrast, is immensely important; it is the sum of one's aspirations, decisions, activities, projects and human relationships.

If this is accepted, then this means that there are certain acknowledged conditions in which life has less value than others. The ANP may need to explain to parents that there are some conditions that are incompatible with life, such as anencephaly and trisomy 18. In cases such as these, where life is accepted by many as having no value, termination may be morally justifiable. In such cases abortion may be viewed as being preferable to bearing a live neonate who instinctively struggles but inevitably fails to survive. The outcome of abortion or live birth will be a fatality, and killing a fetus within the womb is thought to be less traumatic to parents than a live birth followed by death.

Linking abortion with economics

There is also an economic issue linked to termination for fetal abnormalities of which the ANP should be aware. This relates to the intense medical and social interventions required by a child with severe disability. The ANP, whose agenda will always put patients rather than economics as priorities, may find this an issue that is morally unpalatable. However, health economists realize that the birth of a handicapped child entails a significant future burden of care to the health service, social services and the family. Any proposed screening programme to detect congenital defects will be scrutinized on the basis of cost benefits. Is this a euphemism whereby abortion is advocated because handicapped children are deemed to be too expensive? It may be argued from a perspective of social justice that using economics to justify the decision of terminating pregnancies that would otherwise result in handicapped children is appropriate because it allows for allocation of resources to other deserving cases (Chapple, 1994).

Screening in pregnancy

The ability to diagnose an increasing range of fetal abnormalities during pregnancy has been heralded as a great achievement within obstetrics. Many ANPs working within midwifery may themselves conduct screening tests that are designed to highlight potential abnormalities. However, screening tests in pregnancy may be viewed as an attempt to produce only perfect babies. This could signify an element of eugenic manipulation within our society, as suggested by Sutton (1990, p. 14):

The logic behind selective abortion and prenatal diagnosis with a view to abortion of fetuses affected by illness or malformation, is the logic of negative eugenics.

Eugenics is generally recognized as immoral. The tragic perspective of carrying a child with an abnormality is, however, also recognized. The link between aborting an abnormal fetus and the ethos of creating perfect human beings is undeniably close – perhaps a little too close for comfort. It is pertinent to remember that Hitler started his history of atrocities by legalizing abortion. Is the justification for abortion on the grounds of fetal abnormality the first step towards creating a super-race, or should the advances of medical technology be welcomed without question? It may be the ANP's place to ensure that staff contributing to screening programmes in pregnancy, together with clients undergoing these procedures, have thought these issues through.

Making ethical dilemmas real

In order to examine further those ethical issues relating to abortion for fetal abnormalities it is appropriate to consider specific conditions that may be detected antenatally. Chromosomal abnormalities are readily detected and these are responsible for causing various syndromes, of which Down's syndrome is probably the most well known. This is an abnormality in chromosome 21, and is manifest by low IQ and altered physical appearance; 50 per cent of affected individuals also have congenital heart defects. However, the degree of mental retardation is variable. Reciprocal translocations can occur whereby some of the (number 21) chromosomes will be affected yet others will be normal, and this produces a 'mosaic' pattern. The extent to which these individuals will be affected is therefore impossible to gauge. Many terminations are performed for babies affected with Down's syndrome, yet how can this be justified when there is such variance in the condition and in associated quality of life?

Down's syndrome is one of the more severe chromosomal abnormalities. There are many other abnormalities that may occur. These include Klinefelter's syndrome (47 chromosomes – XXY), which occurs in 1 in 1000 males. The affected individual will be eunochoid and infertile, will develop gynaecomastia, and will have a decreased IQ (specifically a 10–20 point reduction in verbal skills); characteristically there is accompanying shyness and emotional immaturity. Would this constitute a condition that justifies abortion?

Another chromosomal abnormality that may occur is the double-Y syndrome. This is present in 1 in 800 males, causes tallness and high fertility, and results in minor mental illness. There is a particularly high incidence of this condition in tall criminals who undergo genetic testing. Could this condition also be justified as a reason for abortion? If it is argued that it could (for, after all, it is a chromosomal abnormality), then is this not a statement to say that deviant individuals are not wanted in society? If men with double-Y syndrome are renowned for being fertile, then is it right to allow them to reproduce and risk subsequent similarly affected progeny? It is disturbing to see that this argument has led to the supportive quote from Hitler's manifesto, *Mein Kampf* (Hitler, 1925), as no-one could endorse the atrocities that resulted from his views:

> *The demand that defective people be prevented from propagating equally defective offspring is a demand of the clearer reason and if systematically executed represents the most humane act of mankind.*

An alternative view of abortion

The issue of abortion for fetal abnormality may also be seen in terms of preventing parental suffering and making parents' future lives easier. It would be callous to consider this without recognizing that for most potential parents the decision to opt for abortion does not leave them unscathed. The ANP will recognize that abortion is sometimes requested through a genuine compassion for the unborn child itself. The role of the ANP is not only to support parents throughout their decision-making process, but also to provide subsequent support for parents through the process of bereavement and grief for their lost child. The ANP will recognize that, with few exceptions, parents love their unborn children, and the decision to terminate their life can be extraordinarily painful.

If it is considered natural to behave in a way that serves one's own best interests, then abortion may be seen as acting in accordance with nature (Andrews, 1993) when abortion is in the mother's own best interest.

Established ethical viewpoints relating to abortion

The deontological view of abortion is the extremist, 'absolute' view. This view argues that the fetus has a moral right to life and therefore has a right not to be killed. The traditional deontologist believes in the sanctity of life principle, and thus opposes all abortions. This view has a strong religious basis and sees the conceptus as an innocent being, unable to protect itself and therefore deserving our support. The principle of non-maleficence would also be upheld within this view, whereby no harm is done to the fetus. The deontological view incorporates a strong belief in duty and recognizes the duty of the parents to bring up their handicapped child in the belief that good will arise from this. This view, whereby the fetus' right to life is absolute, overrides any conflicting rights such as the mother's right to terminate the pregnancy. However, if a deontologist upholds the absolute principle of autonomy and freedom of choice, then this would support the option of abortion.

Utilitarianism contrasts with the principle of rights. The utilitarian view adopts the principle of the greatest happiness for the greatest number, as outlined by Bentham (1748–1832), and therefore seeks to increase pleasure for all. If a handicapped baby were envisaged as bringing endless problems and sacrifices rather than pleasure, the utilitarian would consider it wrong not to abort an abnormal fetus. However, if a handicapped baby were envisaged as bringing special rewards and a sense of commitment and caring, then the utilitarian approach would argue to maintain a pregnancy with an abnormal fetus. The utilitarian stance sanctioned by John Stuart Mill (1773–1836) argued that sometimes individuals have a duty to sacrifice their own greatest good for the good of others. If this were applied to the abortion dilemma, utilitarianism would advocate observance of a general rule to terminate all malformed fetuses. Yet the idea of making a woman have an abortion against her will has no moral principle to uphold it.

Summary

ANPs will frequently need to promote the autonomy of their patients. It is here, in respecting an individual's autonomy, that the ANP is most likely to be at peace with the issue of abortion. If the ANP accepts that rational individuals should be respected as autonomous decision-makers, they are therefore capable of judging what is right for themselves. However, some would argue that the principle of autonomy also specifies that the actions chosen by an individual should not violate the moral interest of others. Abortion could be seen to be doing just this, unless the concept of mother and baby is seen as a joint entity. Mother and fetus co-exist, united by a bond of love into one special being. If this concept is accepted, then the mother could be seen as having the right to decide what her child would want – life with a disability, or no life at all.

Key points

- ANPs working in primary care or midwifery are ideally placed to support antenatal mothers who discover their unborn child has an abnormality that may justify termination of the pregnancy. Skills in counselling, together with medical knowledge and experience of supporting individuals through life crises, enable ANPs to provide optimum care.
- In order to support women in this situation, ANPs need to have considered all the ethical issues surrounding abortion for fetal abnormality. This will enable them to guide mothers through the moral complexities that lie in store, and is likely to assist in the mother coming to terms with her decision.
- Abortion raises many questions, including the value of life, the issue of personhood, and the rights of individuals. Abortion for fetal abnormalities raises the question of 'what is normal', and carries a threat of eugenic influence. The justification of abortion on the grounds of fetal handicap can be interpreted as undermining the worth of handicapped people. In legal terms the fetus has a weak position, and this means that it is vitally important to clarify its moral worth.
- The extent of parental suffering is easy to ignore within a cold discussion of abortion, yet this suffering must not be forgotten or underestimated. The decision to have an abortion for fetal handicap is ultimately the mother's decision – medical opinion may guide her, but cannot force her. The role of the ANP in this setting is to empower the mother to make a decision that she can live with for the rest of her life.
- If the fetus and mother are seen as one, then this partnership can be viewed as capable of deciding whether or not abortion is justifiable within a particular circumstance. The ANP will need to respect this ethical autonomy.

References

Andrews, J. (1993). Abortion and contraception. In: *Ethics: Aspects of Nursing Care* (V. Tschudin, ed.), pp. 1–32. Scutari Press.

Brody, B. (1975). *Abortion and the Sanctity of Life: A Philosophical View.* MIT Press.

Chapple, J. (1994). Screening issues – the public health aspect. In: *Prenatal Diagnosis: The Human Side* (L. Abramsky and J. Chapple, eds), pp. 54–69. Chapman and Hall.

Fitzpatrick, F. (1988). *Ethics in Nursing Practice: Basic Principles and their Application*. The Linacre Centre.

Garrett, C. and Carlton, L. (1994). Difficult decisions in prenatal diagnosis. In: *Prenatal Diagnosis: The Human Side* (L. Abramsky and J. Chapple, eds), pp. 86–105. Chapman and Hall.

Glover, J. (1977). *Causing Death and Saving Lives*. Penguin.

Harris, J. (1985). *The Value of Life. An Introduction to Medical Ethics*. Routledge.

Hitler, A. (1925) *Mein Kampf*. Introduction by D. C. Watt, English translation by R. Manheim, 1969. Hutchinson.

Johnstone, M. J. (1994). *Bioethics: A Nursing Perspective*, 2nd edn. W. B. Saunders/Bailliere Tindall.

Kenyon, E. (1986). *The Dilemma of Abortion*. Faber and Faber.

Noonan, J. T. (1970). Abortion is morally wrong. In: *Life and Death. A Reader in Moral Problems* (L. P. Pojman, ed.), pp. 269–75. Jones and Bartlett.

Rachels, J. (1986). *The End of Life*. Oxford University Press.

Sutton, A. (1990). *Prenatal Diagnosis: Confronting the Ethical Issues*. The Linacre Centre.

Thiroux, J. (1995). *Ethics. Theory and Practice*, 5th edn. Prentice Hall.

Thomson, J. J. (1971). A defense of abortion. *Philosophy Public Affairs*, **1(1)**, 47–66.

Tooley, M. (1983). *Abortion and Infanticide*. Clarendon Press.

Warren, M. A. (1973). The personhood argument in favor of abortion. In: *Life and Death. A Reader in Moral Problems* (L. P. Pojman, ed.), pp. 304–13. Jones and Bartlett.

Warren, M. A. (1977). Do potential people have moral rights? *Can. J. Philosophy*, **7(2)**.

Wells, C. (1989). 'Otherwise kill me': marginal children and ethics at the edges of existence. In: *Birthrights: Law and Ethics at the Beginnings of Life* (R. Lee and D. Morgan, eds), pp. 195–217. Routledge.

Wertheimer, R. (1971). Understanding the abortion argument. In: *The Rights and Wrongs of Abortion* (M. Cohen, T. Nagel and T. Scanlon, eds), pp. 23–51. Princeton University Press.

Ethical considerations in childhood immunizations for the advanced nurse practitioner

Maria Kidd

Introduction

This chapter aims to discuss the ethical considerations of the childhood immunization programme in the United Kingdom, which will be discussed with reference to advanced nursing practice. There is a wide variation as to what different people consider to be advanced practice. For the purpose of this chapter, advanced practitioners are considered to be those practitioners who think and function at a more in-depth level, regardless of the qualifications they have achieved. As health visitors are thought by parents to be an important source of information regarding childhood immunization (Gill and Sutton, 1998), particular reference will be made to advancing their role. However it is also hoped to raise the awareness of ethical issues concerning immunizations amongst other health professionals who are involved with this programme. In order to consider the ethical issues raised by mass childhood immunization programmes, the principles of autonomy, beneficence and non-maleficence will be discussed.

The ethics of public health issues

There are many ethical considerations in the public health arena. It has been suggested that ethics of public health issues can in some ways be more complex than with therapeutic interventions (Cribb, 1997). With health-promoting activities it is the health professional rather than the client who initiates the contact, whereas usually in a therapeutic situation it is the client who seeks the consultation with a health professional – which implies a willingness on the client's part to participate in the outcome or therapy suggested, as they desire to be 'cured'. In health promotion, the issues are avoidance of potential problems or diseases. Immunization is a prime example of this; it may be perceived to be potentially beneficial rather than giving an actual benefit, as it is not inevitable that a child would contract the disease.

The balance of achieving the greater good for the greatest number of people needs to be weighed against the wishes of the individual, and within health visiting this can create a conflict of interest. A major role of the health visitor is to be involved with public health, and hence consider the needs of the community as a whole (Cowley, 1996; Lynch, 1997). However, health visitors also have a duty to provide care to individual clients and their families (White, 1998). Horner (1998) acknowledges this ethical dilemma of the conflict between the needs of the individual and those of the community, which he considers to be inherent in the domain of public health. In order to practise ethically, health visitors look to the *Code of Professional Conduct* (UKCC, 1992) to inform their judgement, which clearly states that nurses 'serve the interests of society'. However it also requires the practitioner to 'safeguard and promote the interests of individual patients and clients'. Health visitors need to explore ways of balancing their responsibilities between the wider community and those individuals with whom they work and serve. Applying this to the immunization programme, the health visitor needs to balance the need for 'herd immunity', so decreasing the prevalence and spread of disease, against the right of individuals to decide if they wish to participate in such a programme.

The immunization programme is considered to be one of the most successful public health measures amongst children (Bedford and Elliman, 1998). However, for continued efficacy of this programme high uptake of immunization is imperative so that 'herd immunity' can be achieved (DoH, 1996). This reflects a utilitarian stance, whereby it is seen to produce the maximum benefit for the majority of people in society. Tadd and Tadd (1998) concur with this approach, suggesting that in recent times there has been an overemphasis on individualism, and that a more utilitarian approach needs to be considered concerning health issues. Beauchamp and Childress (1994) would also agree that occasionally respect for autonomy may be overridden to benefit the greater good of others. This appears to be a somewhat paternalistic approach, assuming that the 'doctors know best', and that they will subsequently act in the best interests of their patients. The individual has their freedom to choose compromised by paternalism. In the USA this paternalistic approach has been adopted, and immunizations are compulsory as a pre-school requisite. This is not the case in the UK; individual parents are able to make a free choice and are entitled to decline immunizations, thus exercising their autonomy.

Patient autonomy

Seedhouse (1998) suggests that autonomy is at the heart of health care, and as such is at the centre of his 'ethical grid'. Autonomy is described as the capacity to think, decide and act on the basis of such thought and decision, freely and independently (Gillon, 1985). The concept of patient autonomy is protected by the doctrine of informed consent (Aveyard, 2000). For consent to be autonomous, the person needs to be in receipt of full information regarding the procedure that is to be undertaken. This is borne out by the Patients' Charter (NHS Executive, 1995, p. 4), which states that all individuals have the right:

> . . . to be given a clear explanation of any treatment proposed, including any risks and alternatives, before deciding whether to agree to that treatment.

If full information is not given then the consent obtained is not valid, and the person's autonomy is not maintained. However, the person not only needs to be in receipt of that information, but also to be mentally competent enough to comprehend it and to be able to act upon it.

In the case of childhood immunizations, or consent to any treatment of children, the child is not generally considered to be able to make a rational decision. The Children Act (DoH, 1989) clearly states that an individual with parental responsibility may consent to treatment on behalf of the child until he or she reaches the age of majority. However, it also necessitates that the maturity of the individual child is taken into consideration when making decisions regarding care or treatment. This is particularly pertinent in the case of 16–18-year-olds, who may consent to treatment if they are considered to be competent. However, as the immunization schedule currently commences at 2 months old, when a child is obviously not in a position to decide, the decision is made by the parent or guardian on the child's behalf. Therefore, in the case of consent of children, the parent exercises autonomy on behalf of the child.

As already suggested, for autonomy to be maintained it is implicit that consent is informed. However, with regard to immunization, implied consent is generally the accepted principle (DoH, 1996). In other words, it is assumed that the parent is consenting to the immunization merely by attending with the child for an immunization appointment and exposing the injection site on request (Mayon-White and Moreton, 1997). However, caution needs to be exercised in this situation. It may be that the parent is attending in order to ask further questions and discuss the immunization programme before making a final decision as to whether or not the immunizations are considered to be in the child's best interests. In addition, implied consent, even if it is absolutely valid, does not negate the need or responsibility for the provision of unbiased and accurate information. Merely attending for an appointment does not guarantee informed consent.

Mayon-White and Moreton (1997) feel that immunization requires consent to be informed and not merely implied. For this to be the case, the health visitor needs to impart full information regarding which immunizations are being given, the benefits this will offer the child, the risks associated with the immunizations and any side effects that may follow. It is hoped that once parents have considered all the information they have been given, they will make decisions that they consider are in the interest of their child. If the risks have not been explained and the parents give consent, then there could be an action against the attending professional for breach of duty of care in relation to the information given (Diamond, 1995) – in other words, the health professional involved has been negligent in gaining consent, the parent's autonomy has been compromised, and so the consent is invalid. However, there can be occasions when parents are in agreement for their child to have immunizations and clearly do not wish to be given all the facts. It can be difficult to impart additional information when they feel that what they know is sufficient. It could be suggested that any decision made would not be autonomous if they were not in receipt of the full facts. Conversely, giving them information against their will could also be seen as disregarding their autonomy. This poses a dilemma for the health professional.

It has been established that for autonomy it is necessary for people to have sufficient knowledge and understanding on which to base their decision (Seedhouse, 1998). When asking parents to consider immunizations, it is the responsibility of the health visitor to ensure that they are given sufficient information regarding the benefits and risks of such a programme. It is when considering the benefits and risks that the ethical principles of beneficence and non-maleficence can come into conflict.

Beneficence and non-maleficence

Beneficence is a positive moral obligation to do good or act for the benefit of others (Beauchamp and Childress, 1994). Nurses are expected to extend beneficence to the clients they care for. The UKCC *Guidelines for Professional Practice* (UKCC, 1996) state that nurses should:

> . . . *act always in such a manner as to promote and safe guard the interests and well being of patients and clients.*

It is clear that there are many benefits to immunizations, and so there are several reasons why they are considered to be important (Mayon-White and Moreton, 1997). Immunizations offer protection for individuals from infectious diseases that may cause serious illnesses, resulting in significant morbidity or carrying a risk of mortality. Also, outbreaks and epidemics of diseases can be avoided. By achieving 'herd immunity', individuals who have 'genuine' contraindications to immunization, such as immunosuppressed children, should also be protected from disease (Mayon-White and Moreton, 1997). Finally, world-wide eradication of lethal diseases may be possible. This has already been achieved with smallpox (DoH, 1996) – although it has been suggested that the decrease in smallpox has been more to do with improved nutritional status and social conditions than immunization (Pilgrim and Rogers, 1995).

One of the aims of mass immunization stated in the document *Targets for Health for All* (WHO, 1985) was the eradication of poliomyelitis, measles, neonatal tetanus, congenital rubella and diphtheria by the year 2000. By 1996–1997, Britain had already achieved a rate of 94 per cent of children being immunized by their second birthday (DoH, 1997), well on line for achieving the targets. The incidence of diphtheria, haemophilus meningitis, measles, polio, pertussis, congenital rubella and tetanus has greatly reduced in Britain, and much of this has been attributed to the immunization programme.

The latest mass immunization campaign in the UK is against meningitis C. Although this disease affects less people than other meningitis strains, the mortality associated with it is greater. From July 1998 to July 1999, group C meningococcal disease accounted for 150 fatalities amongst 1530 cases (Donaldson *et al.*, 1999). The vaccine was introduced in November 1999, and by June 2000 the number of cases of meningitis C within the immunized groups had fallen by 75 per cent (DoH, 2000), which appears to be very encouraging. However, this is a brand new vaccine and criticism has been levelled that the vaccine has not been trialled for a long enough period of time. On the other hand, it has been argued that although the vaccine itself is new, its constituents have all been included in previous vaccines without causing harm (Glennie, 1999).

Traditionally, health promoters, health care professionals and governments have considered immunizations to be safe and effective (Pilgrim and Rogers, 1995). However, with immunizations, as with any intervention, there are associated risks, and these need to be balanced against the benefits. It is here that the principle of non-maleficence needs to be considered. Non-maleficence is embodied in the phrase 'above all, do no harm', which is commonly attributed to Hippocrates. Beauchamp and Childress (1994) describe it as the moral obligation not to inflict harm. This clearly applies to nursing, and is reflected in the *Code of Professional Conduct* (UKCC, 1992), which states that the nurse must:

> . . . *ensure that no action or omission on your part, or within your sphere of responsibility, is detrimental to the interests, condition or safety of patients and clients.*

The act of immunization itself causes pain and distress for the child and for the parents. However, apart from the issue of inflicting pain on a small child, there are serious considerations (such as the safety of the vaccines and their side effects) that need to be taken into account.

Since the reduction in the number of cases of the diseases it appears that many people, particularly parents, have become increasingly concerned regarding the safety of vaccines (Chen and Destefano, 1998). One aspect of this may be because parents do not see or hear of children suffering from these diseases and the serious complications that may ensue (Baird, 1997), as the diseases are now more rare, whilst a case of vaccine damage to a child is widely reported.

Safety

In an attempt to ensure the safety of vaccines, there are strict criteria regarding their development and licensing. They are also 'prescription-only medicines', and thus their use must be regulated (DoH, 1996). Mayon-White and Moreton (1992, p. 2) state:

> *There is a careful assessment of predictable risks in comparison with foreseeable benefits to the population, and within that assessment is the overriding concern of the interests of the individual subject.*

Extensive trials are conducted whilst vaccines are in development, which consider their safety and efficacy.

There have been several scares over the years, reported in the media, regarding the safety of immunizations. In the 1970s, there were reports connecting the pertussis vaccine with brain damage (Gangerosa *et al.*, 1998). More recently, in 1998, there was much media coverage and public concern when the *Lancet* published a report by Wakefield *et al.* (1998). The media reported that the paper suggested a link between the measles, mumps and rubella (MMR) vaccine and Crohn's disease and autism. However, in the conclusion Wakefield *et al.* stated categorically: 'We did not prove a link between MMR vaccine and the syndrome described' (Wakefield *et al.*, 1998, p. 641). Latterly it has been suggested that autism often presents itself at a similar age to the administration of MMR, but that this is coincidental rather than a causal link (Nicoll *et al.*, 1998). Since then, other research has been published which has failed to find a causal link between MMR vaccine and autism (Taylor, 1999a). However, despite reassurances from the government (DoH, 1998) and health professionals, there followed a fall in coverage of the MMR (Communicable Disease Report, 1998). Many parents were sceptical about the government's reassurances regarding the safety of the MMR. This is maybe not surprising in the light of other health scares, such as *Salmonella* in eggs in the 1980s (Galbraith, 1989). In this case the government was initially dismissive of claims regarding potentials links with ill health, and subsequently produced health warnings regarding eggs. However, as with many scares, once the media coverage decreases the concerns lessen, and in the intervening period the rate of uptake of MMR vaccine is slowly increasing (Communicable Disease Report, 2000).

The meningitis C campaign, which started in November 1999, has not been without its problems. The Department of Health was brisk to respond to safety concerns expressed in the media that the vaccine had been causing meningitis, stating that the vaccine could not cause meningitis because it was not a live vaccine (DoH, 2000).

There is increasing competition in the media, which inevitably leads to sensationalism. Begg *et al.* (1998) pointed out that the media were all too quick to highlight negative findings, rather than focusing on positive features of health campaigns. Journalism has a part to play in public health issues, but Flaysakier (1990) feels that stricter ethical guidelines within the media professions need to be considered, in an attempt to avoid issues being handled unprofessionally.

Side effects

Aside from the concerns regarding the safety of the various vaccines, there are the side effects that can occur following vaccination. It could be argued that all drugs have side effects; and a simple glance at the current *British National Formulary* (1999) would confirm this. However, most drugs are given as treatments, rather than for preventable measures. Side effects from a treatment maybe considered more acceptable, if alleviation of symptoms from a disease is achieved. It maybe difficult for parents to accept side effects when they only see immunization as a potential, rather than an actual, benefit.

The side effects of immunization are well documented (DoH, 1996). In the majority of cases these are mild, including slight pyrexia and localized redness and swelling around the injection site. Unfortunately, there are cases when the side effects can be very serious and have long-term implications for both the child and parents, but these risks are considered to be minimal (DoH, 1996). This minimal risk from immunization may be acceptable to a health care professional; however, it is understandable that parents may not find even a small risk acceptable when considering their own child's health (Richardson and Webber, 1995). What is a minimal risk? Health professionals are provided with information from the Department of Health, which it could be suggested is biased in favour of immunization and does not present the full picture. The incidence of serious side effects is not stated, only the fact that they are rare. In fact no incidence of this 'minimal' risk appears to be cited by any source of information regarding immunization. This poses a problem, as without complete and accurate information parents cannot make an informed decision.

Other concerns

Several other areas of concern have also been highlighted with regard to immunization. One of the criticisms that Pilgrim and Rogers (1995) suggest is that there is 'substantial physical intrusion into a healthy body'. They feel that it is preferable for the body to acquire natural immunity, whereas with immunizations the immune system is deliberately activated to initiate a 'disease response' situation. It is thought that this may have long-term side effects on the immune system, possibly causing iatroganic problems such as auto-immune disorders and cancers (Pilgrim and Rogers, 1995).

Another concern is that of the reality of benefit. It has been suggested that the downward trend in rates of infectious disease was greatest prior to immunization programmes (Pilgrim and Rogers, 1995), and can be attributed to social factors such as clean water supplies. This is certainly a factor in many diseases. However, where immunization rates have fallen there have been increases in the rates of disease (Yarwood and Bozoky, 1998). This has been experienced in Russia, where falling immunity rates have resulted in a diphtheria epidemic (Thompson, 1995). A positive example of changes in epidemiology has been seen following the introduction of the *Haemophilus influenzae* type b (Hib) in 1992. High uptake rates were achieved, and there has been a dramatic decline in this disease (Bowen-Morris, 1997).

The role of the advanced nurse practitioner

As highlighted in this chapter, the immunization issue is an emotive one, with strong feelings being rife amongst some groups within the population (Baird, 1997). It has been established that parents glean information from various sources with regard to childhood immunizations, including health visitors and other health professionals, friends and family, and the media (Gill and Sutton, 1998). It is therefore not surprising that when concerns are raised by any of these sources parents will consider them when making a decision. This can make it difficult for parents to make a truly autonomous decision (Baird, 1997). It is the role of the health visitor not only to give information, but also to allow time for parents to ask questions and discuss their concerns and anxieties regarding immunization. It has been established that full disclosure of the facts is imperative for consent to be informed. In order to give complete information, all possible risks and benefits need to be discussed. This is one area where the principle of veracity or truthfulness can be applied. With the advent of more openness and honesty, the issue of veracity is more evident. The *Code of Professional Conduct* (UKCC, 1992) suggests that nurses must 'work in an open and co-operative manner with patients, clients and their families'.

When discussing the side effects of immunization, how often are all the possible side effects given? More often it is the common side effects, along with appropriate advice as to how to deal with them, that are discussed (Baird, 1997). However, Gill and Sutton (1998) found that 42 per cent of parents wanted more information about immunization, particularly relating to the long-term risks and side effects. Leino-Kilpi *et al.* (1993) concur that clients have greater satisfaction when more information is given to them. Another study found that an increasing number of parents expressed a degree of dissatisfaction with some aspect of the immunization visit (Yarwood and Bozoky, 1998). This would suggest that adequate information is not being given to parents. It has been suggested that there is a bias in the information given to parents (Pilgrim and Rogers, 1995). Parents tend to be given Health Education Authority booklets, such as *Birth to Five Years*, and the health professional's information is predominantly gleaned from *Immunization against Infectious Disease* (DoH, 1996). However, the parent has a right to expect impartial and accurate information from the attending care giver (Sampson, 1998), and it is therefore the responsibility of health visitors to ensure that they are in possession of current knowledge regarding immunizations.

It is imperative that the health visitor does not use persuasion or covert coercion when raising the issue of immunization with parents, in order that they can make an autonomous decision regarding whether or not their child is immunized (Richardson and Webber, 1995). This is especially true when there is increasing pressure on health care providers to meet immunization targets (Richardson and Webber, 1995). Achieving targets is rewarded by financial incentives, and if patients decline immunizations the targets may not be achieved, leading to a subsequent reduction in income. There have been documented cases where general practitioners have had patients removed from their list when they have refused immunizations. This financial incentive may lead to health professionals putting pressure on parents to have their children immunized, and practitioners need to be mindful of this.

If the parent chooses to refuse immunization, even if the health visitor feels that the decision is misguided, this decision must be respected in order to maintain and respect the parent's autonomy. This is reinforced by the *Code of Professional Conduct* (UKCC, 1992), which states that nurses must:

> *recognise and respect the uniqueness and dignity of each patient and client, and respond to their need, irrespective of their ethnic origin, religious beliefs, personal attributes, the nature of their health problem or any other factor.*

It is the health professional's responsibility to support parents who are making their autonomous decision to consent to treatment on behalf of their children, or to refuse such treatment (Taylor, 1999b). Consider the following scenario, which illustrates this point.

Mr and Mrs B's first child died at just over 4 months old of Sudden Infant Death Syndrome (SIDS); this was 5 days following his third immunization. Despite there being no link between immunizations and Sudden Infant Death Syndrome, Mr and Mrs B have always attributed his death to the immunization because of the timing of the death. Since that time they have had another boy who is now 3 years old, for whom they have declined immunizations. Now they have a third child, another son, and again they do not wish him to be immunized. When the health visitor was conducting the primary visit and the subject of immunization was raised, Mrs B immediately began to defend their position of declining immunizations. The previous health visitor had been supportive of their decision not to immunize; however, they had felt pressurized by the general practitioner, who had cited the fact that there was no link between Sudden Infant Death Syndrome and immunizations. The health visitor has a dilemma. There is no evidence to suggest a link between Sudden Infant Death Syndrome and immunization. However, as far as these parents are concerned they perceive there to be a link, which in the light of their experience is understandable. The parents feel that the potential benefits of immunization are greatly outweighed by the prospect of a further child dying. The risk of the two surviving children in this family contracting any of the diseases against which immunization offers protection are probably minimal due to the effects of herd immunity. In order for the health visitor to maintain the autonomy of these parents, their decision was respected. The parents were reassured by the health visitor that their point of view was understood, and also that their decision would not have a negative impact on any other care which they would receive.

It can be difficult for individuals to assert their rights in an issue such as immunization, when mass immunization is a policy that is so widely accepted both at a national and international level. For this reason, it is imperative that parents are supported in their decisions.

Summary

Parents are constantly making decisions regarding their children in everyday life. However, decisions regarding medical interventions such as immunizations can be overwhelming (Taylor, 1999b), and it is the responsibility of the health visitor to ensure that the information provided to the parents is detailed, accurate and up-to-date to allow the parents to make an informed decision. A balanced view of the benefits and side effects needs to be given. If full information is not given, then the health visitor could be accused of paternalism or possible negligence; if persuasion and coercion are used, the parent's autonomy will be compromised.

There remains a dilemma for the health visitor who is endeavouring to maintain the autonomy of the individual whilst also considering the greater good of the community. There is no easy solution to this problem, but an increased awareness of the ethical principles of autonomy, beneficence and non-maleficence will guide the health visitor's thinking and actions, subsequently enhancing the practitioner's thoughts and moving him or her towards advanced practice.

Key issues

- The parent's autonomy must be maintained by obtaining informed consent.
- Parents need to be given information that fully discusses the benefits and the risks of immunization.
- Parents need to have adequate opportunities and time to discuss their feelings and concerns regarding immunizations.
- It is the professional's responsibility to ensure that he or she keeps up to date regarding new developments within the immunization programme, and carefully to consider these developments.
- Parents need to be supported when making what can be difficult decisions on behalf of their children with regard to immunizations, and at times this will involve the health professional acting as advocate for the parents.

References

Aveyard, H. (2000). Is there a concept of autonomy that can usefully inform nursing practice? *J. Adv. Nursing*, **32(2)**, 352–8.

Baird, A. (1997) Ethics of immunization. *Practice Nursing*, **8(3)**, 16–18.

Beauchamp, T. and Childress, J. (1994). *Principles of Biomedical Ethics*, 4th edn. Oxford University Press.

Bedford, H. and Elliman, D. (1998). *Childhood Immunization: A Review*. Health Education Authority.

Begg, N., Ramsay, M., White, J. and Bozoky, Z.(1998). Media dents confidence in MMR vaccine. *Br. Med. J.*, **316**, 561.

Bowen-Morris, J. (1997). Protection against Hib: study shows that immunization policy is a success. *Health Visitor,* **70(9)**, 344–6.

British National Formulary (1999). Number 38. London, British Medical Association & Royal Pharmaceutical Association of Great Britain.

Chen, R. and Destefano, F. (1998). Vaccine adverse effects: causal or coincidental? *Lancet,* **351**, 356–61.

Cribb, A. (1997). Ethics: from health care to public policy. In: *The Challenge of Promoting Health* (L. Jones and M. Sidell, eds), pp. 236–59. Open University Press.

Communicable Disease Report (1998). *MMR Coverage,* **8**, 39.

Communicable Disease Report (2000). *COVER Programme: July to September, 1999,* **10**, 34.

Cowley, S. (1996). Health visiting and public health. In: *Community Health Nursing. Frameworks for Practice* (Gastrell and Edwards, eds), pp. 272–84. Balliere Tindall.

Department of Health (1989). *The Children Act.* HMSO.

Department of Health (1996). *Immunization against Infectious Disease.* HMSO.

Department of Health (1997). *Vaccination and Immunization, Summary Information for 1996–97, England.* HMSO.

Department of Health (1998). MMR vaccine is not linked to Crohn's disease or autism. Press release98/109, 24 March.

Department of Health (2000). The safety of meningitis vaccine. Public Health Link/CMO's urgent communication. CEM/CMO/2000/8.

Diamond, B. (1995). *The Legal Aspects of Child Health Care.* Mosby.

Donaldson, L., Moores, Y. and Howe, J. (1999). *Introduction of Immunization against Group C Meningococcal Infection.* Department of Health.

Flaysakier, J. (1990). The journalist as a health educator. In: *Ethics in Health Education* (S. Doxiadis, ed.), pp. 93–106. Wiley & Sons.

Galbraith, N. (1989). Chicken and egg. *Br. Med. J.,* **297**, 704.

Gangerosa, E., Galazka, A., Wolfe, C. *et al.* (1998). Impact of the anti-vaccine movement on pertussis control: the untold story. *Lancet,* **351**, 356–61.

Gill, E. and Sutton, S. (1998). Immunization uptake: the role of parental attitudes. In: *Immunization Research: A Summary Volume* (V. Hey, ed.), p. 26. Health Education Authority.

Gillon, R. (1985). *Philosophical Medical Ethics.* Wiley & Sons.

Glennie, L. (1999). Know your enemy. *Community Practitioner,* **72(11)**, 350–51.

Horner, S. (1998). Ethics and the public health. In: *Ethical Issues in Community Health Care* (R. Chadwick and M. Levitt, eds). Arnold.

Leino-Kipli, H., Iire, L., Suominen, T. *et al.* (1993). Client and information: a literature review. *J. Clin. Nursing,* **2**, 331–40.

Lynch, U. (1997). Public health: the way forward. *Health Visitor,* **70(5)**, 194–5.

Mayon-White, R. and Moreton, J. (1997). *Immunizing Children.* Radcliffe Medical Press.

NHS Executive (1995). *The Patient's Charter and You.* Department of Health.

Nicoll, A., Elliman, D. and Ross, E. (1998). MMR vaccination and autism. *Br. Med. J.*, **316**, 715–16.

Pilgrim, D. and Rogers, A. (1995). Mass childhood immunzation: some ethical doubts for primary care workers. *Nursing Ethics*, **2(1)**, 63–70.

Richardson, J. and Webber, I. (1995). *Ethical Issues in Child Health Care.* Mosby.

Sampson, D. (1998). Immunization: identifying and resolving the ethical issues. *Community Practitioner*, **71(4)**, 133–5.

Seedhouse, D. (1998). *Ethics: The Heart of Health Care.* Wiley & Sons.

Tadd, W. and Tadd, V. (1998). Concepts of community. In: *Ethical Issues in Community Health Care* (R. Chadwick and M. Levitt, eds), pp. 6–15. Arnold.

Taylor, B. (1999a). Autism and measles, mumps and rubella vaccine: no epidemiological evidence for a causal association. *Lancet*, **353**, 2026–9.

Taylor, B. (1999b). Parental autonomy and consent to treatment. *J. Adv. Nursing*, **29(3)**, 570–76.

Thompson, J. (1995). Facts, fiction and fears. *Health Visitor*, **68(7)**, 292–3.

United Kingdom Central Council (1992). *Code of Professional Conduct.* UKCC.

United Kingdom Central Council (1996). *Guidelines for Professional Practice.* UKCC.

Wakefield, A., Murch, S., Linnell, A. *et al.* (1998). Ileal-lymphoid-nodular hyperplasia, non-specific colitis and pervasive developmental disorder in children. *Lancet*, **351**, 637–41.

White, E. (1998). Ethical dilemmas: a solution for community nursing. *Community Practitioner*, **71(3)**, 100–102.

World Health Organization (1985). *Targets for Health for All.* WHO.

Yarwood, J. and Bozoky, Z. (1998). Prevention through immunization: take the evidence-based approach. *Practice Nurse*, **16(4)**, 216–18.

Informed consent and the advanced nurse practitioner

Kate Stuart

Introduction

In the course of their everyday work nurses are confronted with a multitude of ethical issues, and one particular area that provides daily challenges for health care workers is that of informed consent. This may be in relation to minors, unconscious patients or those with mental health problems, to name but a few. It would therefore seem essential that nurses have a clear understanding of what informed consent is, and of some of the complex legal and ethical issues surrounding it.

The issues surrounding this subject are too many to allow discussion of them all here, and indeed some, such as the consent to participate in research and consent in minors are major topics in their own right. However, consent will be considered in relation to ethical principles and theories, as well as the position in the eyes of the law. Also, because from both a legal and an ethical stance the concept of competence is central to informed consent, it will be discussed in some detail, taking into consideration some of the dilemmas facing doctors, nurses and other health care professionals. This will focus particularly on issues related to consent that may arise in relation to the A&E department and the developing role of advanced nurse practitioners (ANP).

The majority of the literature on informed consent refers to doctors, but with the increasingly overlapping roles of doctors, nurses and other health care workers, much of the previous literature can today be considered to apply to all health care professionals.

Informed consent and ethical theories and principles

It is quite possible to give consent to an examination or procedure without any knowledge of what it entails. Informed consent aims to provide individuals with information and knowledge that allows them to make an informed choice. The United Kingdom Central Council for Nursing and Midwifery, in their document *Exercising Accountability* (UKCC, 1989), described informed consent in the following way:

> *It is self evident that for it to have any meaning consent has to be informed . . . 'informed consent' means that the practitioner involved explains the intended test or procedure to the patient without bias and in as much detail (including detail of possible reactions, complications, side effects and social or personal ramifications) as the patient requires. In the case of an unquestioning patient the practitioner assesses and determines what information the patient needs so that the patient may make an informed decision.*

Although this has now been superseded by *Guidelines for Professional Practice* (UKCC, 1996), the new document does not mention the need for lack of bias. This must surely be an important factor in informed consent, and is one that has not always been considered both in nursing and in the traditionally paternalistic medical profession.

Informed consent has its foundation in the two ethical principles of autonomy and truth telling. Autonomy can be regarded as ' . . . the individual's freedom to decide her or his goals and to act according to those goals' (Faulder, 1985, p. 23). Individuals must be provided with the knowledge to make a balanced choice regarding their care, based on their personal values, goals and beliefs. By ensuring this, the practitioner demonstrates respect for them as autonomous beings. However, unless the principle of truth telling or veracity is also upheld the patient may be unable to make an informed choice due to inaccurate (or lack of) information, and therefore be deprived of the right to autonomy (Thompson *et al.*, 1994). Denying the principle of veracity risks destroying the relationship between health care professional and patient, which is based on a foundation of trust.

Knowledge of ethical theories and their application can help in understanding the dilemmas surrounding informed consent. Jeremy Bentham (1748–1832) and John Stuart Mill (1806–1873) are the two philosophers most commonly associated with the theory of utilitarianism. The main principle of this theory is often described as that of 'the greatest happiness for the greatest number', reflecting the fact that both Bentham and Mill were hedonists. In their view, the rightness of an action is dependent upon its consequences, resulting in only one absolute moral rule – the promotion of utility. However, there are flaws in this theory; Grassian (1981) gives the example of slavery, claiming that at the time it may have been justified by maximizing the happiness of the majority, although most people today would condemn the practice. Additionally, if the slaves were in the majority, then the concept of providing the greatest happiness for the greatest number would no longer be true.

As a rule, the National Health Service (NHS) can be said to work to a utilitarian framework, attempting to use the resources available to provide the best health care possible for the majority of the general public. For example, the NHS finds it hard to justify providing a multi-organ transplant to one recipient when the individual organs could be used to improve or save the lives of several recipients.

In direct contrast to utilitarianism is the theory of deontology or duty ethics, associated with the philosopher Immanuel Kant (1724–1804). Kant was more concerned with the motives for people's actions, as opposed to the consequences of them. He believed that actions should be based on moral duty and not on the pursuit of happiness, which he considered could lead to grave injustices. Justice was central to Kant's belief in people as rational beings; that each deserves respect and should have the opportunity to set his or her own goals, providing these do not interfere with the freedom of others. Kant devised a single principle to explain his view of morality, called the 'categorical imperative'. This requires individuals to act according to rules that they would wish to become a universal law. For the deontologist, individuals are seen as an end in themselves and they should never be treated as a means to an end by others.

Health care workers who work on the concept of individualized patient care reflect Kant's ideas. His belief in people as rational beings deserving of dignity and respect, with the capability to make their own choices, is central to autonomy and informed consent in the NHS.

The level of informed consent obtained from an individual may depend upon whether the health care professional (or organization) works according to utilitarian or deontological beliefs. Take, for example, the man who requires surgery for a particular problem. The traditional method is very invasive and painful, leaves a large scar and has a long recovery period. There is, however, a newer method, which is far less invasive but involves advanced and highly expensive technology. It also leaves minimal scarring and recovery is rapid. A professional with utilitarian beliefs may not consider the new method to be an option, as the expense may deprive others of treatment. Therefore, he explains the traditional method, answering the patient's questions, but does not mention the alternative treatment. Conversely, the deontologist would not consider the expense of the new treatment to be a deterrent, believing that there is a moral duty to inform the patient of all the options available. However, the deontologist may also make the patient aware of the possible consequences to others should he or she choose the newer treatment.

Types of consent

There are three main types of consent. The first is *implied consent*, and occurs in many contacts between practitioners and their patients. An example is when patients roll up their sleeve for the nurse to take their blood pressure. There may be no verbal exchange, but by their actions there is implied consent to the procedure. The second type of consent is *verbal consent*. Again this can be a perfectly valid type of consent, and is commonly used for simple procedures. It entails the practitioner gaining verbal permission from the patient to carry out the procedure. However, the MDU (1996) and the UKCC (1996) both recommend that details should be recorded in the patient's notes. Both of these types of consent are used daily by nurses.

The final form of consent, *written consent*, is in the main used by doctors; however, with the ever expanding and developing role of nurses, this situation is changing. Written consent is not normally legally essential, but does provide documentary evidence that consent has been obtained. It provides some evidence that a meeting has occurred between the patient and the individual obtaining consent, but is no guarantee that the consent was informed or that information provided to the patient was correct. There are, however, three circumstances where written consent is a statutory requirement (Dimond, 1994); these relate to abortion, the use of gametes and embryos, and specific circumstances when giving treatment for mental health disorders.

Studies have shown that junior doctors are obtaining consent for procedures about which they have inadequate knowledge (Houghton *et al.*, 1997; Mulcahy *et al.*, 1997), making it unlikely that consent was adequately informed. Although it is not disputed that the ideal person to gain consent should be the individual who is to carry out the procedure, it would seem more appropriate for an advanced nurse practitioner with a high level of specialist knowledge and clinical expertise to gain informed consent than a junior doctor with inadequate knowledge.

Indeed, an increasing number of complex and invasive procedures may be carried out by the ANP that definitely necessitate them gaining the clients informed consent themselves.

It is important to bear in mind that gaining a patient's consent, be it implied, verbal or written, does not mean that it was 'informed consent'. In order for consent to be valid and informed, the following factors should be adhered to (adapted from Jones, 1995; MDU, 1996):

1. It must be voluntary and not obtained by coercion.
2. It should be obtained before the procedure begins and before any form of sedation is given.
3. Whenever possible, it should be obtained by the person who will perform the procedure. Where this is not possible, consent must be obtained by someone who is suitably qualified and knowledgeable regarding the details and risks of the procedures and any alternatives. Patients must be given adequate information, set at a level and in language appropriate to them, so that they are fully aware of what they are consenting to.
4. The patient must be capable of understanding the procedure.

Informed consent and the law

According to the law, adults who have the capacity (competency) to consent to treatment also have the right to refuse treatment, even if that should endanger their lives. This is reinforced by Gilberthorpe (1996, p. 41), who states that:

> Society and the law demand that patients' autonomy be respected by their physicians, even if the physicians themselves may not always feel that this is consistent with best medical practice or, indeed, in patients' best interests.

Thompson *et al.* (1994) emphasized three points about patients' rights (and human rights in general) that can be related to informed consent:

1. Having rights does not mean that one must exercise them
2. The existence of rights does not mean that there are not limits to them
3. Negative expressions of the right (i.e. the right to refuse treatment) are in general, much more controversial than positive expression of those rights.

These points will be discussed in this chapter.

Within civil law there are two main torts (recognized civil wrongs) that are used in connection with informed consent; the torts of battery and negligence. Battery can be described as any physical contact without consent, and in theory could be applied to merely touching a patient without consent, irrelevant of whether any harm occurred or if the treatment was beneficial. However, in reality this is unlikely to occur, and it is most likely to be applied when a treatment or procedure has been carried out without consent, even if the practitioner felt it was in the best interests of the patient. Take for example the case of Devi *v.* West Midlands AHA (1981), where Mrs Devi consented to a minor gynaecological operation but the surgeon, on finding that she had a ruptured womb, sterilized her. She won her action of battery, as she had not consented to sterilization.

There have also been instances where cases of alleged battery have been brought to court claiming that the doctor concerned did not tell the patient of the risks of an operation or procedure, therefore making their 'informed consent' invalid. Chatterton *v.* Gerson (1981) and Sidaway *v.* Board of Governors of the Bethlem Royal Hospital (1985) were both such cases. Miss Chatterton and Mrs Sidaway were both left disabled after operations and claimed that they had not been told of the risk of such injury. Both claimants lost their cases, with the judges stating that their consent was valid as long as the procedure had been explained to them in broad terms. The judges also suggested that such cases should be brought as negligence as opposed to battery (Dimond, 1995).

These rulings would lead us to believe that if patients have given consent to a procedure but believe that they were not given adequate information to make an informed consent, then they may action the tort of negligence. In order to win a negligence case, 'a patient must prove that, on the balance of probabilities, injury resulted from the negligent act of the doctor' (BMA, 1992). However, within English, law these actions have frequently been unsuccessful, as the case of Blyth *v.* Bloomsbury AHA (1993) demonstrates. Mrs Blyth, who was a nurse, suffered prolonged bleeding after being given a contraceptive injection. She had asked questions about her treatment, but was still given inadequate information about the potential side effects of the drug. The trial judge ruled in Mrs Blyth's favour but was overruled by the Court of Appeal, who believed that the information Mrs Blyth had received was consistent with current medical practice at the time.

The outcomes of these cases can be related to what has become known as the *Bolam test*, developed from the case of Bolam *v.* Friern

Hospital Management Committee (1957). Mr Bolam suffered from a manic depressive disorder and, as a result of a course of electro-convulsive therapy, suffered severe pelvic fractures. His reasons for suing the hospital were that although he had consented to treatment, he was not informed of the inherent risks or that these could be minimized by the use of constraints or muscle relaxants. Justice McNair, who presided over the case, made it clear that a doctor:

> *. . . is not guilty of negligence if he has acted in accordance with the practice accepted as proper by a reasonable body of medical men skilled in that particular art . . .*

At the current time, cases of alleged negligence are likely to be measured against this standard. However, a concern about this ruling is that a defendant doctor may produce expert witnesses who back his actions and render him not liable for negligence, even if the majority of doctors would have acted differently. Seemingly, the Bolam test acts more in favour of the doctor than of the patient bringing the case.

As the ANP role remains very much in its infancy, and due to the blurring of the boundaries of the role with the traditional medical role, ANPs are likely to be judged according to the Bolam test should they find themselves in court. Where they find themselves performing procedures that were previously carried out by doctors they are likely to be judged according to the standards expected of a junior doctor or possibly a registrar, depending on the circumstances.

The law differs greatly in Australia and many states of the USA, where informed consent is based on a patient-oriented standard of disclosure. In 1992 the High Court of Australia adopted this approach during the case of Rogers v. Whitaker, declaring that:

> *The law should recognize that a doctor has a duty to warn a patient of a material risk inherent in the proposed treatment: a risk is material if, in the circumstances of the particular case, a reasonable person in the patient's position, if warned of the risk, would be likely to attach significance to it or if the medical practitioner is or should be aware that the particular patient, if warned of the risk, would be likely to attach significance to it.*

This patient-oriented approach to informed consent is far more in keeping with the concept of individual autonomy. It also reflects Kant's categorical imperative, for if the Bolam test were to become universal law, practitioners who became patients themselves could expect no more information than the average doctor would consider to be necessary. However, under the patient-oriented standard of disclosure, they could expect to be given the depth and amount of information that, as individuals, they would require in order to make an informed decision. The dilemma that does arise, however, is just how much information to give. Meisel and Kuczewski (1996) are concerned that some physicians, unsure of the amount of information to disclose to their patients, end up by providing every last detail, which, according to eminent psychologist Richard Lazarus (1979), has a risk of being detrimental to the patient. This is surely a situation where common sense and good communication skills prevail.

The patient-oriented standard depends on practitioners having some knowledge of their patient, in order to make a judgement as to how much information an individual is likely to require. In an Accident and Emergency department (A&E) it can be difficult to gain adequate knowledge of individuals because most of them are in the department for a short time. This is an area where ANPs have a strong advantage, for their role encompasses both medical and nursing care of their patients. Consequently they spend longer with patients and have a greater opportunity to build up relationships and gain knowledge of individuals than either the doctors or other nurses, and are therefore better placed to provide the information that the patient needs to make an informed decision. In the UK, the dilemma of how much information to give to a patient also exists, but due to the legal stance there is perhaps more risk of being given too little information than too much.

Consent can be viewed as both an emotional and a rational process for practitioners and patients (Alderson, 1995). Practitioners may be tempted to withhold information that they believe patients will find too distressing to cope with, and consequently be unable to make rational decisions. This can be justified in terms of the *therapeutic privilege*, which allows them to withhold information under precisely such circumstances. However, Meisel and Kuczewski (1996) emphasize that this should not be abused simply because the practitioner is unable to deal with passing on unpleasant and painful information to a patient, or because the information may result in the patient refusing consent to treatment that the physician considers to be vital. Although genuine use of the therapeutic privilege is made by physicians from a stance of non-maleficence, it is still paternalistic – particularly as the information being withheld is, almost without exception, of great significance to the patient concerned (Faulder, 1985).

Difficulties can arise when health professionals hold differing opinions as to what information should be given to the patient. For example, a doctor may have obtained consent from a patient, providing a level of information that would adhere to the Bolam test. The nurse caring for that patient may believe that the patient has a right to more detailed information, which could perhaps include alternative treatments available, and that without this additional information the patient will not be able to give fully informed consent.

Competence

We have already highlighted the factors that need to be present for consent to be valid, but there is still the problem of the patient's capacity to consent. The Medical Defence Union defines a competent adult as (MDU, 1996, p. 9):

> *. . . a person who has reached 18 years of age and has the capacity to make treatment decisions on his own behalf. Capacity is present if the patient can fulfil the following criteria:*
> *1. Comprehend and retain the treatment information*
> *2. Believe that information*
> *3. Weigh that information in the balance to arrive at a choice.*

The competency of those under the age of 18 years and their capacity to consent is a complex issue that will not be addressed here.

As a rule, the person making the decision as to the patient's capacity is the doctor who is caring for that person, although there are times when this decision may be left to the courts. Nurses also make these decisions each time they carry out a procedure or treatment on a patient, although they are probably not conscious of having done so. In their developed role, ANPs should possess a heightened awareness of the criteria related to a patient's capacity. They must also possess the ability to articulate clearly why they feel a patient does or does not have the capacity to consent to treatment. As with any new role, ANPs will be carefully observed by other professionals to see how they respond to such challenges.

Several concerns are raised regarding the health care professional who makes the important decision regarding a patient's capacity, for an inaccurate assessment of a patient's ability to consent may deprive them of the basic right to autonomy. The decision may be influenced by several factors, including the communication skills of the practitioner concerned. The patient's ability to comprehend the treatment information will often depend on the language used. It is not uncommon to witness a practitioner who is unable to speak at a patient's level of understanding and resorts to the use of medical jargon. Faulder (1985) believes that class divisions also are the cause of some communication barriers between doctor and patient. Are these patients then denied their right to make decisions about their treatment because of the practitioner's inability to communicate? Again this is an area where the ANP can be invaluable, as highly developed communication skills are a key factor of the role. By taking sometimes complex medical procedures and explaining them in simple, layman's terms, ANPs are able to act as advocates for patients by allowing them to make choices they may otherwise have been denied.

In today's multicultural society, communication difficulties occur when there is a language barrier. If patient and practitioner are unable to speak the same language, how can it be possible to determine a patient's capacity? Even if relatives are present to translate (and these can often be children), there is the risk of receiving their biased interpretations of the patient's replies. In a reversal of the situation, the practitioner's command of English may be poor so that the patient has problems understanding the explanation of the treatment. The risks here are that the practitioner assumes incorrectly that the patient has given informed consent, or concludes that the patient does not have the capacity to consent and so acts in his or her 'best interests'. In these cases, access to a good translation service is the most effective way of ensuring that a patient has the capacity to consent.

Medicine has by tradition been paternalistic in nature, believing that doctors know what is best for their patients. Nursing too has shown paternalistic tendencies and, although the introduction of holistic and individualized care has done much to reduce this, it is still in evidence at times. How many nurses have not felt frustration or even annoyance towards patients who discharge themselves from their care, refusing treatment that could be considered to be in their 'best interests'? As long as the nurse has ensured that the patient is competent and has made an informed choice, then the nurse's obligations to the patient have been fulfilled. Practitioners must be aware that, unbeknown to them, there may be past or current circumstances in a patient's life experience that influence the decisions made.

Paternalism is in direct conflict with autonomy and informed consent, and there must be some concern over whether a patient whose decision does not agree with that of the doctor is deemed to be incompetent. Take the case of Re. T (1992), a 20-year-old pregnant woman whose refusal to consent to a blood transfusion was overruled by the courts. The grounds for this ruling were that the patient, who was not a practising Jehovah's Witness, had only made this decision after a visit from her mother, who was a committed Jehovah's Witness. It was considered that the patient had been put under undue pressure from her mother. There are two ways to view this situation: first, that the courts were wrong in removing her right to refusal of treatment when there was no concrete evidence to show that she was incompetent; and secondly, that the decision to refuse treatment had only been made because of the pressure from her mother and the patient may have been relieved that the decision had been taken out of her hands. When discussing this particular case, Stauch (1995, p. 162) remarked that:

> *By separating the capacity to make a treatment decision from the rationality or otherwise of that decision, we appear to give proper weight to the autonomy of the individual. The alternative, allowing choice but then discounting those choices adjudged to be irrational, seems equivalent to giving the patient no real choice at all.*

Stauch comments further that the approach in Re. T appeared to be beneficence-based, addressing the patient's 'best interests' as opposed to encouraging patient autonomy. Health care professionals have to accept that patients do at times make what they may later consider to be wrong decisions, but that does not mean that they should be considered to have reduced capacity.

Paternalism also raises the issue of power. The skills and expertise that doctors and nurses possess give them a great deal of power over their patients, who are vulnerable and dependent (BMA, 1988). Utilization of these skills to make the best decisions for their patients has been the basis of the traditional beneficent paternalism of the NHS. By providing patients with knowledge, practitioners are handing over a degree of this power and going some way to redressing the unequal relationship between practitioner and patient (Alderson, 1995). However, concerns arise if some practitioners are reluctant to relinquish this power and attempt to retain control by withholding information or declaring patients to be incompetent and therefore unable to make their own choices. ANPs who feel comfortable with their own knowledge and clinical skills and readily pass that knowledge on to others will have a different power base. Their power comes from their ability to empower patients and allow them to make informed, knowledgeable choices about their health care.

It should be remembered that there will always be patients who, although perfectly competent, choose to have their practitioner make health care decisions for them. These people have decided 'autonomously to abdicate their autonomy' (Seedhouse, 1988), but this does not mean that they do not want informing about their care. It would seem wise on the practitioner's behalf, before fully accepting this choice, to explore the issue further to ensure that there is not an underlying problem that has not been addressed. It may be that the patient does not understand the information but feels too embarrassed to ask, or perhaps he or she is one of the many adults with limited literacy skills and may have been given written information. Certainly within a busy A&E department this is an ideal role for ANPs. They will often not have a specific patient workload, and may find it possible to take the necessary time and skills to address these issues. Choosing to have their practitioner make health care decisions for them does not mean that patients have given up the right to be informed. These patients also maintain the right to reassert their autonomy in decision-making at any time, should they so choose.

The patient's 'best interests'

If a patient has been found to lack the capacity to consent to treatment (whether for the right or wrong reasons), then the practitioner is expected to act within the 'best interests' of the patient. However, it could be questioned how many of them really make a decision based upon the views of the patient. Artnak (1997, p. 62) comments that:

> ... an assessment of what is good and right for the patient has historically been based on a medical model intent on preserving life and relieving suffering.

This reflects the ethical principles of beneficence (doing good) and non-maleficence (doing no harm), and certainly appears to be the correct basis from which to plan an incompetent patient's care. However, the patient's concept of what is good and right may be in complete conflict with that of the health care professionals, being based not on the medical model but on religious beliefs, life experience, social situation etc.

The BMA and Law Society (1995) consider that assessment of a patient's capacity to consent requires the practitioner to have knowledge of the individual that includes their cultural values and social situation. It seems reasonable then that decisions about a patient's 'best interests' should also require this level of knowledge. The MDU (1996) refers to a checklist of factors pertinent to deciding the patient's 'best interests' as recommended by the Law Commission (1995, p. 44):

1. *The ascertainable past and present wishes and feelings of the person concerned, and the factors that person would consider if able to do so.*
2. *The need to allow and encourage the person to participate, or to improve his ability to participate as fully as possible, in anything done for and any decision affecting him.*
3. *The views of other people who it is appropriate and practicable to consult about the person's wishes and feelings, and what would be his best interests.*
4. *Whether the purpose for which any action or decision is required can be as effectively achieved in a manner less restrictive of the person's freedom of action.*

How many practitioners ensure that they have this knowledge (or indeed feel that it is necessary), and how practical a task is it for them to achieve? In situations where there is only brief contact with a patient, as in an outpatient setting or an A&E department, this presents the ANP with a particular challenge. It is unrealistic to expect practitioners to have enough knowledge of such a patient to be sure that the patient makes a decision that is in his or her own best interests. In order to reach as balanced a decision as possible the ANP should consult with all those caring for the patient (BMA and RCN, 1995), including relatives and significant others, and design a plan of care that it is hoped reflects what the patient would have chosen if competent.

Consent in emergencies

The A&E department provides a multitude of dilemmas relating to informed consent and refusal. From the patient's perspective, loss of autonomy through feelings of helplessness, lack of control and knowledge has been shown to be an overriding concern of patients attending A&E (Byrne and Heyman, 1997). Informed consent should help to reduce these concerns.

If an unconscious patient is admitted to the A&E department and requires lifesaving treatment, it is generally accepted (and may be seen as part of the duty of care) that health care professionals will intervene to save the patient's life and carry out any treatment that it would be detrimental to the patient's health to delay (Fletcher *et al.*, 1995). Any practitioner who acted in these circumstances, providing they showed due care and skill, would be immune from liability should a case of battery or negligence arise (BMA, 1992). However, care that could safely wait until the patient was able to consent should not be given.

There may be times when things are not so clear-cut. Consider the following scenario. A young male who has been involved in a road traffic accident is brought by ambulance to the A&E department. Due to severe blood loss he is unconscious and urgently needs a blood transfusion, but a relative accompanying him informs staff that the patient is a Jehovah's Witness and would not want a transfusion. There are two options. The first is to take this into account and give only non-blood products. However, there is no certainty as to the accuracy of the information from the relative regarding the patient's wishes. The alternative is to give a blood transfusion on the basis that not to do so would put the patient's life at risk, and that legally a relative is unable to consent or refuse consent for an adult.

If, however, as in the Canadian case of Malette *v.* Shulman *et al.* (1988), the patient had on his person a signed card stating specifically that in an emergency he did not wish to be infused with any blood products due to his beliefs as a Jehovah's Witness, justifying ignoring this directive would be extremely difficult. Giving blood in these circumstances would be to override a patient's autonomy and, as Wreen (1991, p. 125) states:

> Not to respect an autonomous person's refusal of treatment when that refusal is religiously based is not to respect him as a person at the deepest level, the level at which he has tried to reconcile himself to the limitations of his own human existence.

This is a situation where ANPs would utilize their knowledge of ethical issues and the law to act as an advocate for the patient and guide the health care team to an acceptable solution.

Some patients may be fully competent on initial admission to A&E but during their time there become incompetent – perhaps by losing consciousness. This can provide practitioners with dilemmas. Consider, for example, a patient who has taken a drug overdose in a suicide attempt, but has specifically stated that he does not want any treatment. He is fully aware of the possible consequences of refusal of treatment and appears to have made a balanced decision; therefore he cannot be deemed to be incompetent. When this patient then becomes unconscious and his life is threatened, are practitioners justified in treating him? This case will be expanded on shortly, but, according to Jones (1995), providing the patient was competent when the decision was made, treatment should not be given and the individual's autonomy respected.

A common problem in any A&E department is the drunk, head-injured patient. What happens if such a patient refuses treatment? A&E staff are faced with the conflict of respecting autonomy and their duty of care to the patient. It could be argued that, due to the effects of alcohol and possibly the head injury, the patient should be considered to be temporarily incompetent. However, from a legal stance it may not be accepted that alcohol has made an individual incapable of consenting to or refusing treatment. If the patient were allowed to leave the A&E department, would the staff be failing in their duty of care and putting themselves at risk of claims of negligence if the head injury was found to be significant? Conversely, would they be assaulting the patient if restraint were necessary for treatment? As with many such issues, there is not a clear-cut and definitive answer. In each situation, the individual circumstances along with a good knowledge of ethical issues and the law are needed to make a balanced decision.

Hunka (1993) tells of an incident in an intensive care unit involving a patient who was himself a doctor, had ensured that he was very well informed of his condition, and had cared for others in similar situations. This gentleman made it very clear on several occasions that if he became critically ill, he did not want 'extraordinary medical therapy' in order to keep him alive. Unfortunately he became critically ill and, despite his very well informed refusal, his son insisted that everything was done for him. He ended up being ventilated for 30 days before he died, despite his express wishes. Hunka (1993) makes attempts to justify this, arguing that belief in the sanctity of life and its preservation was greater than and therefore took preference over the individual's autonomy and rights in relation to the withholding of treatment.

This raises several issues, beginning with the fact that a relative of an adult patient has no legal jurisdiction to consent to or refuse treatment for the patient unless a prior agreement has been made. This was not the case here. It is also argued that it was done in the patient's best interests. However, as the patient had made it very clear what his best interests were, it must be suspected that the best interests being upheld here were those of the son and the medical staff, reflecting Thiroux's statement (Thiroux, 1995, p. 46) that:

> *. . . it is much easier for individuals to know what their own interests are than it is for them to know what is in the best interests of others.*

The argument of non-maleficence is also proposed, but the patient may well have considered that by actively treating him against his wishes the medical staff were in fact doing him harm. Finally, Hunka (1993) puts forward the 'slippery slope' argument, that there is a moral line that should not be crossed – for example, by withholding treatment from this patient it would then be far easier in the future to withhold treatment from patients who are unable to either consent to or refuse treatment. However, this patient was an educated medical practitioner, who was fully competent when he made his decision. He also made his wishes clear to a number of people, both staff and his family. Surely the possibility that in the future a practitioner with dubious moral standards would use this case as a reason to withdraw treatment from a non-consenting, incompetent patient is a poor excuse to override the dignity and autonomy and show such lack of respect for the gentleman in this instance?

Let's expand further on the case of the patient who takes an overdose. A 36-year-old man is brought into the A&E department having taken a large overdose of an opioid-containing drug. On arrival he refuses consent to any treatment, stating that he wishes to die. As the drug takes effect he becomes increasingly drowsy and unresponsive. What action should the health care team be taking at this point? This is always a complex situation, and one to which there seems to be no definitive answer. First, there is the issue of competence to be addressed. It has already been mentioned that if the patient was competent, then his decision must be respected. However, the other side of the argument is, can someone who is distressed enough to attempt to take his own life be considered to have the full capacity to make truly rational choices?

Again, this is a situation where there is no definitive answer. One argument could be that due to his temporarily disturbed mental state and the probable effects of the drug, he should not be considered competent. Therefore, staff should go ahead and treat this patient in a manner they believe to be in his best interests. This action is upheld by the case of F v. Berkshire Health Authority (1989), when it was stated that it is possible for a doctor to provide treatment to an incompetent adult patient provided the doctor believes it to be in the patient's best interests and especially if it is potentially life saving. The case also concluded that involvement of the courts is not always necessary, which is a particularly important addition in A&E care.

In contrast to the above case is that of Re. C (1994), where a known schizophrenic patient refused treatment for amputation of his leg because of progressive gangrene. In this instance the court upheld his refusal of treatment, considering that the patient demonstrated that he understood the nature, purpose and effects of the treatment involved, and the potential consequences of his refusal. The problem with this case in relation to patients in A&E is the time factor. If treatment is potentially life saving, there may not be the time available that is needed to deliberate over situations where competency is unclear. In such situations practitioners would be obliged to perform the life-saving treatment as part of their immediate duty of care, and to reassess the patient's competency when his or her life was out of danger.

Not all issues relating to informed consent are as obvious as those highlighted so far. The existence of ageism is well documented (Hope, 1994; Lookinland and Anson, 1995), as is the relationship between the increased risk of receiving inadequate health care and rising age (BMA and RCN, 1995). Artnak shows particular concern over informed consent and refusal in the elderly, and raises concerns that (Artnak, 1997, p. 61):

The presence of such a prejudice towards older people by those evaluating their medical decisions can cause those decisions to be either modified, discounted, or perhaps altogether ignored because of the age of the person who made them.

The concern must be that there is a risk of decisions being taken for the elderly regarding their care without them ever being assessed as incompetent. This is also reflected in the way that relatives are often given information regarding the condition of elderly patients, without their consent or even before they themselves have been informed. Although probably done with the best intentions, it is overstepping the boundaries of both autonomy and confidentiality. If the patient is deaf or has some difficulty in communicating, there may be a temptation to discuss care with the relatives simply because it is quicker and easier (BMA and RCN, 1995). This is a particular risk in an A&E department, where workload pressure is high or the patient's condition may warrant a sense of urgency. However, unless the patient's condition is life threatening, there is no justification for not taking the time to ascertain the patient's wishes and gain informed consent.

Advanced nurse practitioners are well placed to ensure that informed consent is obtained from older patients wherever appropriate. By spending time with such patients, ANPs are able to establish the best means of communicating with them and providing information regarding their illness or treatment. Due to their knowledge and experience, ANPs are also well placed to intervene if they consider that an individual's autonomy or confidentiality is being violated in any way. If a patient refuses consent, the ANP may be able to establish the reasons why. Is it due to fear, lack of knowledge, or perhaps differing values due to personal life experiences?

Summary

This chapter has given some consideration to the highly complex issue of informed consent. By having an understanding of the ethical theories and principles underpinning the concept, it is easier to comprehend some of the conflicts that arise between the organization, individual practitioners and the legal system. Establishing an individual's competence has shown itself to be a source of concern for many reasons, relating in part to paternalism, communication skills, beneficence, non-maleficence and the best interests of the patient. The A&E department is an area where problems pertaining to consent are frequent occurrences and a selection of potential situations has been discussed, although a number of these are equally applicable to other departments. There are several aspects of informed consent that have not been discussed here, mainly because they are subjects in their own right, and some of the areas that have been discussed require more space than is available here to do them full justice.

The role of ANPs has also been considered in relation to informed consent. Their high level of communication skills, their clinical knowledge and skills and their understanding of ethical and legal issues, combined with their unique position within the health care system, puts ANPs in a strong position to ensure that true informed consent is obtained.

Finally, as informed consent aims to maintain the autonomy of patients it seems appropriate to end with a description of informed consent written not by a health care professional but by a journalist whose intention is to inform the general public about such complex issues (Faulder, 1985, p. 2):

> *Informed consent is about the right to control our own destinies and to determine our own ends as far as is humanely possible; it is about the right to make choices and the right to refuse consent; it is about the right*

*of individuals to preserve their integrity and dignity whatever physical
and mental deterioration they may suffer through ill health; it is about
our duty always and in all circumstances to respect each other as fellow
human beings and persons.*

Key points

- Informed consent is based on the ethical principles of autonomy and truth telling.
- Belief in the ethical theories of utilitarianism or deontology may influence the level of informed consent obtained.
- Gaining a patient's consent does not guarantee that it was informed.
- By law, an adult who has the capacity or competency to consent to treatment can also refuse that treatment.
- Decisions regarding a patient's capacity to consent can be complex and controversial.
- An ANP is often ideally qualified and placed to ensure that true informed consent is obtained.

References

Alderson, P. (1995). Consent to surgery: the role of the nurse. *Nursing Standard*, **9(35)**, 38–40.

Artnak, K. E. (1997). Informed consent in the elderly: assessing decisional capacity. *Seminars Periop. Nursing*, **6(1)**, 59–64.

British Medical Association (1988). *Philosophy and Practice of Medical Ethics*. BMA.

British Medical Association (1992). *Rights and Responsibilities of Doctors*. BMJ Publishing Group.

British Medical Association and The Law Society (1995). *Assessment of Mental Capacity. Guidance For Doctors and Lawyers*. BMA.

British Medical Association and The Royal College of Nursing (1995). *The Older Person: Consent and Care*. BMA.

Byrne, G. and Heyman, R. (1997). Patient anxiety in the accident and emergency department. *J. Clin. Nursing*, **6**, 289–95.

Dimond, B. (1994). *The Legal Aspects of Midwifery*. Books for Midwives Press.

Dimond, B. (1995). *Legal Aspects of Nursing*, 2nd edn. Prentice Hall.

Faulder, C. (1985). *Whose Body is it? The Troubling Issue of Informed Consent*. Virago Press Limited.

Fletcher, N., Holt, J., Brazier, M. and Harris, J. (1995). *Ethics, Law and Nursing*. Manchester University Press.

Gilberthorpe, J. (1996). Some thoughts on consent. *J. MDU*, **12(2)**, 41–3.

Grassian, V. (1981). *Moral Reasoning. Ethical Theory and some Contemporary Moral Problems*. Prentice Hall.

Hope, K. W. (1994). Nurses attitudes towards older people: a comparison between nurses working in acute medical and acute care of the elderly settings. *J. Adv. Nursing*, **20**, 605–12.

Houghton, D. J., Williams, S., Bennett, J. D. *et al*. (1997). Informed consent: patients' and junior doctors' perceptions of the consent procedure. *Clin. Otolaryngol.*, **22**, 515–18.

Hunka, S. A. (1993). The right to refuse treatment – an ethical case study. *Intensive Crit. Care Nursing*, **9**, 82–7.

Jones, M. A. (1995). Ethical and legal responses to patients who refuse to consent to treatment. *Br. J. Urology*, **76(2)**, 9–14.

Law Commission (1995*). Mental Incapacity. Item 9 of the Fourth Programme of Law Reform: Mentally Incapacitated Adults* (Law Com. No. 321). HMSO.

Lazarus, R. S. (1979). Positive denial: the case for not facing reality. *Psychology Today*, **Nov.**, 44–60.

Lookinland, S. and Hanson, K. (1995). Perpetuation of ageist attitudes among present and future health care personnel: implications for elder care. *J. Adv. Nursing*, **21**, 47–56.

Medical Defence Union (1996). *Consent to Treatment*. The MDU Ltd.

Meisel, A. and Kuczewski, M. (1996). Legal and ethical myths about informed consent. *Arch. Internal Med.*, **156**, 2521–6.

Mulcahy, D., Cunningham, K., McCormack, D. *et al.* (1997). Informed consent from whom? *J. R. Coll. Surgeons (Edinburgh)*, **42**, 161–3.

Seedhouse, D. (1988). *Ethics: The Heart of Health Care*. John Wiley & Sons.

Stauch, M. (1995). Rationality and the refusal of medical treatment: a critique of the recent approach of the English courts. *J. Med. Ethics*, **21**, 162–5.

Thiroux, J. (1995). *Ethics: Theory and Practice*. Prentice-Hall.

Thompson, I. E., Melia, K. M. and Boyd, K. M. (1994). *Nursing Ethics*. Churchill Livingstone.

United Kingdom Central Council (1989). *Exercising Accountability. A Framework to Assist Nurses, Midwives and Health Visitors to Consider Ethical Aspects of Professional Practice*. UKCC.

United Kingdom Central Council (1996). *Guidelines for Professional Practice*. UKCC.

Wreen, M. J. (1991). Autonomy, religious values, and refusal of life-saving medical treatment. *J. Med. Ethics*, **17**, 124–30.

List of cases

Blyth *v.* Bloomsbury Health Authority (1993) 4 Med LR 151

Bolam *v.* Friern Hospital Management Committee (1957) 1 WLR 582 (QBD)

Chatterton *v.* Gerson (1981) 1 All ER 257

Devi *v.* West Midland Area Health Authority (1981) Ca Transcript 491
F *v.* Berkshire Health Authority (1989) 2 All ER 545–571
Malette *v.* Shulman (1988) 47 DLR (4th) 18, (1990) 67 DLR (4th) 321
Re. C (adult refusal of treatment) [1994] 1 WLT 290
Re. T (adult refusal of treatment) (1992) 4 All ER 649
Rogers *v.* Whitaker (1992) 109 ALR 625
Sidaway *v.* Bethlem Royal Hospital Governors (1985) 1 All ER 643

The advanced nurse practitioner: empowerment in witnessed resuscitation

Alastair Gray

Introduction

Accident and Emergency (A&E) departments, with their complex mix of the routine and mundane on one hand and human dramas on the other, are often the focus for ethical dilemmas. Such issues range from decisions about prioritizing needs and resources, to the ease with which patients can be 'labelled' by staff, and access (or otherwise) of patients/ relatives to services (Jones and Hall, 1994; Walsh, 1994; Thompson *et al.*, 1996). A current issue of ethical concern focuses on the question of whether relatives should be permitted to be present during resuscitation efforts on a critically ill relative (Redley and Hood, 1996). In the light of the current debate on this subject, this chapter will examine the issues surrounding choice being made available to relatives, and the potential role of the advanced nurse practitioner in facilitating the enactment of relatives' informed choice and in supporting and educating colleagues to enable choice to be offered to relatives.

At the heart of the debate about whether relatives should witness resuscitation events lies a crucial question about harm. Health professionals are clearly expected to use their knowledge and skills for the benefit of patients and carers, and to protect them from harm. However, what constitutes 'harm' and, perhaps more importantly, who decides what is harmful? Common 'wisdom' seems to suggest that witnessing a relative's traumatic resuscitation and subsequent death constitutes harm. However, on the other hand, does denying relatives a choice to be with their loved ones up to the point of death also have the potential to constitute harm? A real-life example may help to illustrate this point. In an article taken from an accident and emergency journal only a few years ago, the anguish of a mother separated from her daughter is poignantly expressed (Gregory, 1995):

I am plagued with the knowledge that I was not with my beautiful daughter as she was dying.

This mother was denied the choice to be with her daughter as she was being resuscitated. It was not impossible to have achieved this, but merely that there was no one to facilitate access, no policy to support it, and no one to act as advocate for this distressed woman. Considering another point of view, what about the patient's perspective? Is it possible that harm is also experienced by the person who is in the process of dying if relatives are kept away? Who decides what is harmful is a very important question, since it gets to the heart of who is in control of the events that surround patients and their relatives' lives.

In reality decisions are made largely by health professionals, who appear to regard themselves as best able to act in the 'best interests' of their patient. This clearly paternalistic stance is exemplified by the phrase 'doctor/nurse knows best' (Thompson *et al.*, 1996). In fact this approach is endemic in clinical practice generally, and even cursory observation reveals that general care processes seldom include a real and active patient/relative role. It is not surprising that this state of affairs is particularly magnified when the decision-making processes involved in care delivery and disease management are examined.

Although anecdotally widespread, it is encouraging that this type of mindset is increasingly being questioned and challenged both by the lay public and, perhaps more importantly, by health professionals themselves.

A professional collaborative model?

Professional codes of ethics are increasingly making reference to the inclusion of the recipients of care, both in the delivery of care and also in the decision-making processes about that care (Clause 5, *Code of Professional Conduct*, UKCC, 1992). Moreover, many leading nurses are at the forefront of the debate calling for the patient/health professional relationship to be a collaborative one, rather than that of the professional taking control. In an empowering relationship the professional offers knowledge, skill and judgement, and the patient or relative considers the potential benefits and risks involved in proposed options for care (Chameides, 1997). What must prevail is the patient/relative perspective of what is best for them. Clearly the principles of beneficence, non-maleficence, justice, autonomy and self-determination are inherent within this dynamic (Seedhouse and Lovett, 1992; Morgan, 1996; Thompson *et al.*, 1996). However, nurses charged with the task of supporting such a process need to be very special people with a broad range of knowledge, skills, attitudes and experience. They must command the respect of colleagues and, above all, be able to influence and change the climate in which care is delivered, for that climate exerts considerable influence on the nature of clinical practice. Such people are rare, but may be found carrying the title advanced nurse practitioner (Manley, 1997; Scholes, 1998).

Witnessing resuscitation versus a culture of separation

Undoubtedly the rise of technical interventions has brought both benefits and problems to patients. This is particularly true in the area of resuscitation processes. Widespread teaching about basic life support encourages members of the public to use those skills and get involved when the need arises. Increasingly it is the case that 'bystanders' may in fact be close family members. However, once health professionals arrive at the scene of a life-threatening drama, relatives tend to be ushered away from the traumatic scene for their 'benefit' (Baskett, 1995; van der Woning, 1997). However, is this really of benefit? There is now growing evidence that relatives would often prefer to be present (Redley and Hood, 1996; Barrat and Wallace, 1998; Meyers *et al.*, 1998). This may actually confer significant benefits (Hanson and Strawser, 1992; Connors, 1996; Eichorn *et al.*, 1996), while harm may occur where access is denied or where relatives are suddenly removed from the scene when the patient deteriorates (Redley and Hood, 1996).

Another clinical example illustrates the point. Imagine the situation where an elderly person's daughter, having found her mother collapsed, commences prompt basic life support. The ambulance arrives and the crew continues the resuscitation efforts. The daughter remains present throughout. On arrival in accident and emergency, daughter and mother are separated, and the daughter is taken to the relatives' room. On asking to be with her mother, she is told: ' . . . it's probably best if you stay here, the resuscitation room is a bit frightening'. Trying to be helpful, the nurse adds, 'We're doing all we can . . .'

It is suggested that such situations are not uncommon. Patients and their carers suddenly find themselves in a frightening, disorientating and often experience profound disempowerment and even zation. Moreover, the essential human characteristics of self-ation and freedom become greatly restricted (Gaylord and Grace, 1995; Thompson *et al.*, 1996). It is not just the health drama into which they are suddenly thrust that has caused this, but also the impact of the unfamiliar rules and restrictions by which health professionals in effect 'control' the environment (Wright, 1996).

An improving situation?

The nature and quality of care given is critically dependent on the attitudes, beliefs and perspectives of the health professional. Moreover, the degree to which the professional's perspectives fit with those of the recipient of care is critical in determining whether patients and relatives needs are met (Ewins and Bryant, 1992). However, Rubin (1996) points to the inability of some, even many, nurses to make a real or 'qualitative' distinction between individual patients/relatives. The inevitable consequence of this is that care offered is reduced to what is 'routine' for that type of condition or problem. In A&E departments, 'structural' issues make this worse, hindering an individual response (Loveridge, 2000). Frequently there are too few staff and too many patients. The need to make rapid assessments and to keep things moving is a high priority, and responding to people as individuals in this context can be challenging to say the least (Tschudin, 1994). Moreover, with the focus on the patient, sight can easily be lost of the attending relatives. Clearly these pressures challenge the very concept of 'personhood' which is intrinsic to each individual, and cut to the very heart of what constitutes ethical behaviour by health professionals (Malone, 1993; Thompson *et al.*, 1996).

In the context of an individual resuscitation event, the quality of staff responses to attending relatives can be legitimately judged by the degree to which the care provided reflects an accurate interpretation and understanding of those relatives' feelings, beliefs and hopes. The manner in which A&E nurses care for both the dying person and their relatives is now widely recognized as significant in determining a family's ability to accept the death and deal with the crisis. While inevitably in critical situations resuscitating a dying person is the priority for staff, this should not prevent effective care from also being provided for attending family members. Not to consider this implies a lack of respect for those suddenly rendered powerless and bereft, and hinders them receiving an effective and adequate response to their need (Seedhouse and Lovett, 1992). The fact that this was recognized as long ago as 1944 by Lindemann (cited by Tye, 1993) and yet until more recent years has often been poorly carried out is puzzling, and rather a sad indictment of the caring professions.

However, it remains that, in recent years, the need for supportive care for attending relatives has received much greater attention (RCN and BAAEM, 1995; Davies, 1997). Significant strides have been made in recognizing that relatives need specific resources and in providing those resources. This is particularly important because it provides the basis for seeing relatives as legitimate recipients of A&E services themselves, and not merely as appendages to their patient–relative (RCN and BAAEM, 1995). However, a simplistic and superficially 'caring' response to this is for relatives to be neatly removed to the sterile environment of a relatives' room, where tea can be administered.

While undoubtedly providing dedicated physical resources is appropriate and beginning to see relatives as worthy recipients of care is welcome, a major barrier remains; the strong, almost instinctive tradition of separating critically ill patients and relatives. This practice flies in the face of growing evidence that when relatives are given sufficient information and support, they are able and want to exercise choices (Adams *et al.*, 1994). Specifically, choices offered to relatives may include whether to enter the situation at all, to remain present when things become difficult, to leave, or to change their minds at any point during the event (Hanson and Strawser, 1992; Redley and Hood, 1996). Simply offering the choice of being with their loved one returns a measure of personal control, even if the relatives' choice is not to be present (Connors, 1996; Meyers *et al.*, 1998). Addressing the issues that uphold the 'doctrine of exclusion' is now the next logical step in improving care for relatives. Before this can be achieved, however, there needs to be an analysis of the reasons for maintaining the practice of denying choice, and also an examination of who is best placed to move forward this advance in care.

The effect of witnessed resuscitation

In seeking to explore this subject and find solutions to the problems that relatives experienced in being excluded from the resuscitation room, American nurses at the Foote Hospital found that selectively allowing relatives into the resuscitation room had a number of benefits (Hanson and Strawser, 1992). However, initially they found that fellow colleagues identified a number of barriers to allowing relatives to witness resuscitation (Hanson and Strawser, 1992), and similar concerns have been highlighted since elsewhere (Adams *et al.*, 1994). Collectively, the major themes include:

1. How would family members react to situations with the potential to distress them further – would they be disruptive or even collapse themselves (Back and Rooke, 1994)?
2. How would staff perform under scrutiny (Resuscitation Council, 1996)?
3. Could staff cope with the extra emotional burden (Saines, 1997), given that the presence of relatives very much reminded them of the 'human-ness' of the situation (Eichorn *et al.*, 1996)?
4. Are staff experienced enough to support relatives, and what sort of support is needed?
5. What are the long-term effects for relatives (van der Woning, 1997)?

It appears that the key thread running through these themes is the need for a particular quality of support and facilitation. For relatives, in all cases the need is for a knowledgeable, compassionate and sensitive professional (Wright, 1999), but specifically within the resuscitation room more is needed. The principal need is for someone who can explain the clinical environment and procedures being carried out in a way that is intelligible. This can be difficult, requiring a clear and in-depth clinical understanding of what is happening, so it can be explained and justified in the heat of the moment (Pullen, 1995; Brummel, 1998). For example, asystole on a cardiac monitor is useful pictorial evidence of a hopeless situation even to the lay person, but what about other cardiac wave forms incompatible with life but which imply activity (Wright, 1999)? Through clear explanation of clinicians' thinking processes, decisions being reached and treatment carried out, support and reassurance can be offered.

A concurrent yet perhaps more difficult role is the feeding back of relatives' perceptions and concerns to the clinical team, both during the event and afterwards during debriefing. A measure of the quality of nursing provided is the degree to which the attending nurse is able to and indeed does take on the necessary role of advocate during such an event (Mark-Maran, 1993). However, are there sufficient people equipped and able to fulfil such a role effectively?

It fact it appears that, in spite of the best intentions of the staff, a large number of patients and relatives continue to depend on what may only be termed 'benign paternalism' (Pullen, 1995). In other words, and for whatever reason, patients and relatives are unable or unwilling to speak for themselves, and instead look to the nurse to speak on their behalf. Beauchamp and Childress (1989), critical of paternalism generally, sanction this form only if harm prevented or benefit achieved outweighs loss of autonomy, the individual's condition prohibits their choice, and the interventions are widely accepted.

A further apparent need for the advocacy role exists when examining relationships between certain principal and other family members. Wright (1996), for example, found that male relatives often spoke on behalf of their younger female relatives, yet were frequently inaccurate in representing their views and feelings. Clearly the needs of all concerned are both multifaceted and not infrequently contradictory, and the role of advocacy is inevitably complex and demanding.

Curtin and Flaherty (cited by Gaylord and Grace, 1995, p. 15) explore the complexity of advocacy in nursing, providing a broader definition:

The nurse–patient relationship is determined by the patient's needs and the nurse's responses to them. The foundation of the relationship is advocacy in the sense that the nurse . . . defends, vindicates, . . . is friendly to, . . . upholds . . . The purpose of the relationship is among other things to maintain or to return control of his life to the patient. However the form of the relationship varies . . . The needs of the patient, the knowledge and ability of the nurse, and environmental circumstances all influence the form of the relationship.

The key issue here is of the health professional being 'other centred' – seeking to put themselves in the relatives' shoes and see things from their point of view (Begley and Blackwood, 2000). Indeed, ultimately autonomy concerns the development of a freely self-chosen and informed plan. Restriction of autonomy through control by professionals is not 'other centred' but 'profession centred', and limits the ability of the recipients of care to formulate a plan and act upon it (Morgan, 1996). It is suggested that it is for expert nursing to minimize the first and maximize the second. Moreover, this needs to take place not merely in individual events, but to pervade the whole climate of emergency services.

Benner (1984), ever the pioneer, takes advocacy a further and important step when she speaks of the need for patients and their relatives to be 'empowered'. Regarding witnessed resuscitation, probably the most extreme example of empowerment is in relation to ultimate decisions about continuing or stopping treatment. This is certainly controversial, but perhaps there is a place for seeking to draw relatives into that decision-making process (Back and Rooke, 1994; Belanger and Reed, 1997). Acting as an advocate (and certainly as an agent of empowerment) is a demanding role, and too much so for many nurses. It is suggested that advanced nurse practitioners are best placed to provide these special roles. The distinct personal characteristics, experience and thorough preparation of ANPs positions them well to act therapeutically and respond effectively to the complexity of human need (Scholes, 1998).

It is clear so far that the dynamics between relatives and health professionals are important, but the prevailing dynamics between professionals exert a critical influence too. It cannot be assumed that common views and beliefs prevail between team members. Consequently, a significant question remains: who can facilitate effective communication and uphold the relatives' needs and wishes while remaining an integral part of the clinical team? Some might point to the experienced accident and emergency nurse as being suitably equipped for this complex role, but is this appropriate? To appreciate the difficulties faced by the health professional designated with the responsibility to act as facilitator and supporter for witnessed resuscitation, interprofessional dynamics require further exploration.

Professional dynamics and the pain of contact

The nature and dynamics of the relationships between health professionals appear to be notable factors in hindering a holistic response to relatives' need in the context of witnessed resuscitation. Medical authority and power is rooted in actual and perceived legal responsibility for decisions about treatment (Thompson *et al.*, 1996). The logical extension of this is that all too easily decisions are based primarily on the views of the medical practitioner 'in charge' of the event, rather than collaborative decisions being reached. The result in this context is that, where it does occur, access by relatives to the resuscitation room is based on *ad hoc* decision making. 'Ultimate decisions' are frequently, even usually, made by medical staff. Decisions are based not fundamentally or primarily on carefully identified relatives' wishes, but on the whim of the senior medic present.

Moreover, specific arguments against allowing access can also be couched in notions of what is 'legal'. It is perhaps easier in complex clinical decision making for the ethical question of what is right or wrong to be reduced to whether it is 'legal' or 'illegal'. This is exemplified by actions reflecting the need for staff to 'cover themselves', irrespective of what may actually be best for the patient or relative. Blanket responses justifying exclusion have included:

- Insufficient time to assess relatives 'suitability' to be present; that there is a theoretical risk of them also collapsing, and the hospital will then be liable for damages
- The relatives may not be who they say they are, exposing the hospital to charges of breaking confidentiality
- It is impossible to predict how things will develop.

Perhaps these apparently plausible 'reasons' for keeping relatives at arm's length hides another motive. The retention of paternalistic control by medics has already been referred too, but this may in reality co-exist or even hide insecurities about how staff may perform under scrutiny. A lack of confidence, fear of exposure and even inadequate training may also be present. This is compounded where nurses lack the confidence or are unable to challenge the *status quo*. The result is inadequate care, which may not only fail to be beneficent but may actually be maleficent too!

However, in case an overly gloomy picture is presented, there have been some very encouraging direct responses to the fears that professional staff expressed in the Foote study (Hanson and Strawser, 1992; Belanger and Reed, 1997; Ellison, 1998). A major feature is a clear difference in perspective between nurses and doctors. Generally, nurses were more willing to involve relatives (Chalk, 1994); medical staff either wanted to exclude or exercise personal control over access (Chalk, 1995; Redley and Hood, 1996; Thompson *et al.*, 1996). Possibly there are issues here to do with the threat of professional 'failure', graphically displayed in failed resuscitation (Saines, 1997). Conversely, the fact that it was nurses who were more open to having relatives present is perhaps due to generally greater experience in interacting with and supporting relatives.

Clearly the urgent need is to move beyond the technical and procedural demands of the situation and to get to grips with the deeper issues that keep practitioners distant from their patients. Only then can skilful interaction with patients and relatives allow understanding of the relatives' perspective of what is happening and what their needs are

(Loveridge, 2000). However, responding to their real need may be a crucial issue, since it brings with it the added dimension of exposure to the potential pain of human contact (Tye, 1993). Johns (1992) ably sets out the problems of professionals being involved, open and authentic with patients and relatives. He argues that it is inherently stressful for staff, and cites Menzies in 1960 and Jourard in 1971, whose work described the variety of psychoanalytical and social processes that have evolved to protect staff from the painful exposure to such human encounters. Limiting contact with distressed relatives and depersonalizing the dead patient by concentrating on procedural and bureaucratic procedures are examples of this (Malone, 1993). The culture of coping come what may does not help dismantle the barriers to therapeutic interventions with the bereaved. Anecdotes of coping in stressful resuscitation procedures among accident and emergency staff abound, with respect given to those who remain cool, calm and detached. Less is heard of the personal distress felt by colleagues as they react to what they have experienced.

Although death is a regular and usually sudden occurrence in A&E departments, it is generally unexpected and remains difficult for staff to cope with (Saines, 1997). It is perhaps not surprising that staff instinctively resist the additional burden of relatives being present during a stressful resuscitation event. Moreover, when relatives are excluded death can be rendered a mere clinical event – the 'human-ness' thus removed, the event can be more easily handled (Malone, 1993). However, sanitizing traumatic events with superficial solutions misses the point of what is required, and denies the professional and ethical responsibilities of the nurse. While generally there is an assumption that nurses strive to move towards an agreement of meaning between their own interpretation of events and that of the relative they are dealing with, this appears not always to be the case. Comments that exemplify simplistic responses include:

. . . it's in relatives' best interests not to witness the event . . .

or:

. . . what they need is a nice cup of tea and a sympathetic nurse . . .

Avoiding offering the choice to be present in the resuscitation room symbolizes a denial of the fundamental caring relationship inherent within effective nursing (Connors, 1996; Meyers *et al.*, 1998). When there is a conflict of perspective the nurse may be unable to facilitate the relative's expressed wishes, and these wishes become subsumed to those of the health professional retaining control of events (Pullen, 1995).

The discussion so far has focused on the perspective of promoting choice, with an emphasis on overcoming the barriers to permitting entry to the resuscitation room. However, this must be tempered by an appreciation that significant problems can occur if due and rapid consideration is not given to understanding relatives' cultural mindset and values. These may predispose them to want to remain absent. Cresci's experience in Southern Italy (Cresci, 1994) is a case in point, where it was observed that there was an apparent cultural mistrust of all things medical, even to the point of physical violence being perpetrated against medical staff seeking to resuscitate the dying! While happily such potentially damaging reactions do not appear to be the norm in either North America (Hanson and Strawser, 1992; Meyers *et al.*, 1998) or the UK (Barrat and Wallis, 1998), the point made is that for every event, each family member must be judged individually.

The needs of relatives are clearly complex, and in particular may well change during the period of a resuscitation event – for instance, a relative who wishes to be present may not be able to face the explicit nature of invasive procedures (Baskett, 1995). It is one thing to witness such things second-hand on television, as much of the population will have done; it is another to witness this first-hand on a parent or spouse (van der Woning, 1997).

In the light of findings and observations that support letting relatives into the resuscitation room, it appears unethical to keep relatives out as a matter of policy (Malone, 1993). However, despite this there does remain an important obstacle to introducing an inclusive approach. This concerns the selection and preparation of those members of staff who will facilitate this process.

Who is best able to support relatives and colleagues?

Certainly experience would appear to be important when determining who is best able to support relatives and colleagues, and intuitive practice arising from that experience would appear valuable in directing decision making by practitioners. Although there is much to support such a perspective, it is evident that this is insufficient on its own. Dewey, in 1960, cited by Dreyfus *et al.* (1996), comments:

> *An expert . . . is set in his ways, and his immediate appreciations travel in the grooves laid down by his unconsciously formed habits. Hence the spontaneous 'intuitions' of value have to be entertained subject to correction, to confirmation and revision, by personal observation of consequences and cross-questioning of their quality and scope.*

Matthews (1993) suggests that as nurses we are too quick to determine what will or won't be upsetting for a relative, imagining that we are the only ones who can deal with the traumas of resuscitation. Rather, what is needed is courage to let the family decide, acting on their own human gut instinct rather than the professional's paternalistic view of what is best (Adams *et al.*, 1994; Gregory, 1995).

A superficial view of advocacy can lead to grounds for conflict between professionals, where the nurse simply speaks 'for the patient' against the team, yet the nurse requires a great deal of integrity to avoid the pitfalls already referred to in this 'paternalistic advocacy' (Pullen, 1995). A number of writers in fact now point to the concept of empowerment as the way forward instead (Gaylord and Grace, 1995); this viewpoint sees relatives in a position to represent themselves.

Accident and emergency nurses, although otherwise experienced, may be ill equipped to meet the diverse and often contradictory needs of patients, relatives and colleagues. Training is certainly appropriate, and the education of staff in bereavement care is firmly on the accident and emergency training agenda (RCN and BAAEM, 1995; Wright, 1996). However, proposals alone do not appear sufficient to equip individual staff to meet the complex issues and dynamics surrounding the introduction of witnessed resuscitation. It is suggested that advanced nurse practitioners working in accident and emergency are best suited to fulfil this complex role. While they are by definition experienced accident and emergency nurses, their role has been expanded to embrace a unique blend of knowledge, skills and attributes, and a particular role and relationship within the clinical team. These facets, refined by higher-level critical thinking and problem-solving skills and complemented by excellent interpersonal abilities, enable ANPs to best facilitate relatives' wishes and act as the interface between them and other health professionals.

Working with and influencing colleagues is also a vital ingredient. Not every accident and emergency nurse carries sufficient respect and authority to speak for change, and this is an essential qualification for facilitating the following:

1. Establishment of a collective philosophy of care (Saines, 1997; Ellison, 1998) that informs and directs all clinical practice

2. Preparation of clear guidelines to regulate family presence at resuscitation (Emergency Nurses Association, 1995; Resuscitation Council, 1996; Morgan, 1997)
3. Introduction of a robust system for staff debriefing, essential for staff well being (Hanson and Strawser, 1992), which facilitates the ventilation of their reactions and feelings (Redley and Hood, 1996); this may be especially difficult initially, when staff may be apprehensive (Hanson and Strawser, 1992)
4. Identification of suitable staff to facilitate the process of enhancing care and empowering relatives (Pullen, 1995).

Tschudin (1994, p. 4) points to a practical approach to reaching ethical conclusions that asks, 'what is happening?', 'what does this mean?' and 'what is the most fitting response?'. Clearly this is not merely about the professionals' or the relatives' perspective, but involves a complex interplay between the two. The advanced nurse practitioner has the necessary role, skills and attributes to support relatives effectively by answering these questions, and is equally best placed to take note of and respond to staff concerns and anxieties. Indeed, an ongoing latter aspect of the role is conducting research that examines patients' and relatives' perceptions of their needs and rights to witnessed resuscitation (van der Woning, 1997).

The final issue: is promoting choice safe?

The final issue surrounding facilitating relatives' presence in the resuscitation room revolves around the question, what are the long-term effects of doing so? Clearly the level of understanding of critical illness by the general public has increased significantly through graphic media exposure to medical emergencies (Adams *et al.*, 1994; Redley and Hood, 1996; van der Woning, 1997). It is suggested that imagination can be worse than reality and is generally considered less manageable (Wright, 1999). On the other hand, actually witnessing a loved one's resuscitation enables a realistic perception that 'all was done that could be done' (Eichorn *et al.*, 1996). Moreover, psychological acceptance and adjustment is often enhanced by being able to say goodbye and touch the person before death (Gregory, 1995). It has also been suggested that family presence may be a help to the critically ill or dying patient, giving the opportunity for family members to whisper encouraging words and provide a physical touch that is supportive and clearly beneficent (Hanson and Strawser, 1992; Malone, 1993; Meyers *et al.*, 1998). Since family members participate actively in every other stage of life, do health professionals have a right to make the choice to exclude them from the last stage (Saines, 1997)?

Summary

It is clear that while bereavement services to relatives in A&E departments are becoming more widespread and improving, there remains room for progress (Davies, 1997). The advanced nurse practitioner is a key member of the A&E team who, by virtue of his or her unique role and attributes, is best placed to facilitate further development of ethical policy and practice – the development of nursing services that move beyond relatively superficial 'tea, sympathy and information exchange' to a more radical therapeutic engagement beyond 'advocacy' and into genuine empowerment. That empowerment facilitates choices, essential when facing the issue of supporting witnessed resuscitation.

If the implementation of witnessed resuscitation is to become a reality, then leadership is urgently required. The advanced nurse practitioner is ideally placed to provide that leadership and support this process. The prize is an ethically sound and fundamentally caring approach to supporting bereaved relatives.

Clearly an action plan is required to move the debate and process of introducing witnessed resuscitation forward in individual A&E departments. The following points highlight the essential aspects of the plan that will enable the facilitation of witnessed resuscitation to be a reality.

Key points

- Current staff attitudes to witnessed resuscitation need to be established.
- A process for dissemination of research findings in order to highlight benefits and respond to staff concerns must be established.
- A balance must be struck between responding to relative need and what can be realistically provided.
- A realistic local policy must be developed for implementing witnessed resuscitation, using research findings and awareness of local culture.

- Key facilitators of witnessed resuscitation must be identified and trained.
- Staff bereavement education must be developed, to include aspects of support for relatives attending patients in the resuscitation room.
- Support and debriefing opportunities following resuscitation events must established for all staff.

References

Adams, S., Whitlock, M., Higgs, R. *et al.* (1994). Should relatives be allowed to watch resuscitation? *Br. Med. J.*, **308**, 1687–9.

Back, D. and Rooke, V. (1994). The presence of relatives in the resuscitation room. *Nursing Times*, **90(30)**, 34–5.

Barrat, F. and Wallace, D. (1998). Relatives in the resuscitation room: their point of view. *J. A&E Med.*, **15(2)**, 109–11.

Baskett, P. (1995). The ethics of resuscitation. In: *ABC of Resuscitation* (M. Colquhorn, A. Handley and T. Evans, eds), p. 72. BMJ Publishing Group.

Beauchamp, T. and Childress, J. (1989). *Principles of Biomedical Ethics.* Oxford University Press.

Begley, A. and Blackwood, B. (2000). Truth telling versus hope: a dilemma in practice. *Int. J. Nursing Practice*, **6**, 26–31.

Belanger, M. and Reed, S. (1997). A rural community hospital's experience with family-witnessed resuscitation. *J. Emergency Nursing*, **23(3)**, 238–9.

Benner, P. (1984). *From Novice to Expert: Excellence and Power in Clinical Nursing Practice.* Addison-Wesley.

Brummel, S. (1998). Resuscitation in the A&E department: can concepts of death aid decision making? *A&E Nursing*, **6**, 75–81.

Chalk, A. (1994). More on family presence during resuscitation. *J. Emergency Nursing*, **20**, 87.

Chalk, A.(1995). Should relatives be present in the resuscitation room? *A&E Nursing*, **3(2)**, 58–61.

Chameides, L. (ed.) (1997). *Pediatric Advanced Life Support*, pp. 11–1–2. American Heart Association.

Connors, P. (1996). Should relatives be allowed in the resuscitation room? *Nursing Standard*, **10(44)**, 42–4.

Cresci, C. (1994). Local factors may influence decision. *Br. Med. J.*, **309**, 406.

Davies, J. (1997). Grieving after a sudden death: the impact of the initial intervention. *A&E Nursing*, **5**, 181–4.

Dreyfus, H., Dreyfus, S. and Benner, P. (1996). Implications of the phenomenology of expertise for teaching and learning everyday skillful ethical comportment. In: *Expertise in Nursing Practice: Caring, Clinical Judgement, and Ethics* (P. Benner, C. Tanner and C. Chesla, eds), pp. 258–68. Springer.

Eichorn, D., Meyers, T., Mitchell, T. and Guzzetta, C. (1996). Opening the doors: family presence during resuscitation. *J. Cardiovasc. Nursing*, **10(4)**, 59–70.

Ellison, G. (1998). Witnessed resuscitation: the relatives' experience. *Emergency Nurse*, **5(8)**, 27–9.

Emergency Nurses Association (1995). Emergency Nurses Association Position Statement: Family presence at the bedside during invasive procedures and/or resuscitation. *J. Emergency Med.*, **21(2)**, 26.

Ewins, D. and Bryant, J. (1992). Relative comfort. *Nursing Times*, **88(52)**, 61–3.

Gaylord, N. and Grace, P. (1995). Nursing advocacy: an ethic of practice. *Nursing Ethics*, **2(1)**, 11–18.

Gregory, C. (1995). I should have been with Lisa when she died. *A&E Nursing*, **3**, 136–8.

Hanson, C. and Strawser, D. (1992). Family presence during cardiopulmonary resuscitation: Foote Hospital Emergency Department's nine-year perspective. *J. Emergency Nursing*, **18(2)**, 104–6.

Johns, C. (1992). Ownership and the harmonious team: barriers to developing the therapeutic team in primary nursing. *J. Clin. Nursing*, **1**, 89–94.

Jones, C. and Hall, G. (1994). The moral problems involved in the concept of patient triage in the A&E department. In: *Issues in Accident and Emergency Nursing* (L. Sbaih, ed.), pp. 150–64. Chapman Hall.

Loveridge, N. (2000). Ethical implications of achieving pain management through advocacy. *Emergency Nurse*, **8(30)**, 16–21.

Malone, R. (1993). The ethics of exclusion and the myth of control. *J. Emergency Nursing*, **19(2)**, 33a–34a.

Manley, K. (1997). A conceptual framework for advanced practice: an action research project operationalising an advanced practitioner/nurse consultant nurse role. *J. Clin. Nursing*, **6(3)**, 179–90.

Mark-Maran, D. (1993). Advocacy. In: *Ethics: Nurses and Patients* (V. Tschudin, ed.), pp. 65–84. Scutari Press.

Matthews, J. (1993). Insignificant others? *Nursing Times*, **89(13)**, 42.

Meyers, T., Eichorn, D. and Guzzetta, C. (1998). Do families want to be present during CPR? A retrospective study. *J. Emergency Nursing*, **24(5)**, 400–405.

Morgan, D. (1996). Respect for autonomy: is it always paramount? *Nursing Ethics*, **3(2)**, 118–25.

Morgan, J. (1997). Introducing witnessed resuscitation in A&E. *Emergency Nurse*, **5(2)**, 13–17.

Pullen, F. (1995). Advocacy: a specialist practitioner role. *Br. J. Nursing*, **4(5)**, 275–8.

Redley, B. and Hood, K. (1996). Staff attitudes towards family presence during resuscitation. *A&E Nursing*, **4**, 145–51.

Resuscitation Council (1996). *Should Relatives Witness Resuscitation?* Resuscitation Council (UK).

Royal College of Nursing and British Association for Accident and Emergency Medicine (1995). *Bereavement Care in A&E Departments: Report of Working Group*. RCN.

Rubin, J. (1996). Impediments to the development of clinical knowledge and ethical judgement in critical care nursing. In: *Expertise in Nursing Practice: Caring, Clinical Judgement, and Ethics* (P. Benner, C. Tanner and C. Chesla, eds), pp. 170–92. Springer.

Saines, J. (1997). Phenomenon of sudden death: Part 2. *A&E Nursing*, **5**, 205–9.

Scholes, J. (1998). Therapeutic use of self: a component of advanced nursing practice. In: *Advanced Nursing Practice* (G. Rolfe and P. Fulbrook, eds), pp. 257–70. Butterworth-Heinemann.

Seedhouse, D. and Lovett, L. (1992). *Practical Medical Ethics*. John Wiley & Sons.

Thompson, I., Melia, S. and Boyd, K. (1996). *Nursing Ethics*, 3rd edn. Churchill Livingstone.

Tschudin, V. (1994). *Deciding Ethically*. Bailliere Tindall.

Tye, C. (1993). Qualified nurses' perceptions of the needs of suddenly bereaved family members in the accident and emergency department. *J. Adv. Nursing*, **18**, 948–56.

United Kingdom Central Council (1992). *Code of Professional Conduct*, 3rd edn. UKCC.

van der Woning, M. (1997). Should relatives be invited to witness a resuscitation attempt? A review of the literature. *A&E Nursing*, **5**, 215–18.

Walsh, M. (1994). A study of the attitudes of A&E staff towards patients. *A&E Nursing*, **2**, 27–32.

Wright, B. (1996). *Sudden Death, A Research Base for Practice*, 2nd edn, p. 18. Churchill Livingstone.

Wright, B. (1999). Responding to autonomy and disempowerment at the time of a sudden death. *A&E Nursing*, **7**, 154–7.

Advance directives – considerations for advanced nurse practitioners

Mary Akufo-Tetteh

Introduction

Medical technology and modern treatments have improved the lifespan of patients, but many people feel that medical intervention is becoming too intrusive. As patients become more knowledgeable about medical technology, treatments and their legal rights, they are more willing and able to make decisions concerning their own care. Consequently issues such as advocacy and patient empowerment are becoming more appropriate and acceptable to the general public and health professionals alike (Savulescu *et al.*, 1998). Social norms in Western society have made the area surrounding the subject of death or the loss of physical and/or mental independence difficult to discuss, and consequently even close friends or relatives are not always aware of the wishes of the terminally ill or unconscious patient (Farrar, 1992). The knowledge that medical interventions may prolong life but reduce its quality is unacceptable to many individuals. As a result of this an increasing number of documents such as advance directives (ADs or living wills), which state the individual's personal wishes in such events as loss of consciousness, are being instigated.

Advance directives are recognized as legal documents in the USA. In some states, government legislation makes it mandatory for physicians to accept and respect the wishes of patients who produce such a document (Goetschius, 1997). In the UK there is much controversy surrounding advance directives; however, many members of the general public wish to use their increased knowledge and autonomy to make provision for their own future (Berghmans, 1998). Health professionals are likely to be asked for their advice concerning the documentation and utilization of advance directives. Historically the general public feels more able to approach nurses than doctors, and they are therefore more likely to be asked for information about advance directives. Advanced nurse practitioners (ANPs) are in the unique position of having increased knowledge and skills and a wealth of experience, a background that should enable them to guide their colleagues and support their patients in health and illness. The autonomous ANP has a personal and professional responsibility to remain aware of the current legal and personal implications of completing an advance directive.

This chapter gives a general overview of an advance directive and its constituents. The history of advance directives is explored, and the variety of ways in which these documents will be appropriate and applicable is discussed. The role of the ANP both in advising patients and in implementing these documents will become clear. Although some emotive issues such as euthanasia will be mentioned, they will not be discussed in detail.

The history of advance directives

Throughout the ages death has been considered to be not only acceptable but also desirable. Men who lived in Ancient Greece were able to approach their Elders and request the right to die. The Elders would hold Tribunals regularly, where each individual request for a peaceful death would be considered and the successful candidate would be presented with a draft of hemlock to end his life (Matzo, 1997). In the Byzantine era (324–1453 AD) physicians abandoned their terminally ill patients, as it was thought to be egoistic of them to believe that they could cure patients whom the gods had already condemned to die (Lascartos *et al.*, 1999). Other societies, such as those in the Fiji Islands or India, encouraged wives to commit suicide after the death of their husbands (Matzo, 1997).

The genocide that occurred during World War II caused some western societies to change their positive view of death and euthanasia. Such changes in a society's attitudes are common and can be easily understood when they are related to the history and structure of the society in which they are found (Freire, 1972). In the USA in 1972, the Euthanasia Education Council produced and circulated a testimony-type document amongst the general public. The document discussed the availability of modern medical interventions, suggesting that such interventions should not be used as a means to prolong life if the quality of such a life was unacceptable to the individual. As a result of this release, public opinion forced the State of California to produce the Natural Death Act 1976, which required physicians to comply with their patients' wishes (Drain, 1993).

The change in British society's attitudes is highlighted by a subtle change in the *Concise Oxford Dictionary* (1964), which originally described voluntary euthanasia as a 'gentle and peaceful death'. Sixteen years later the definition has changed to 'an act of taking life to relieve suffering' (*Concise Medical Dictionary*, 1980). Further changes in the publics' attitude compelled The House of Lords Select Committee on Medical Ethics to release a statement that described euthanasia as 'A deliberate intervention undertaken with the express intention of ending a life to relieve intractable suffering' (House of Lords, 1994).

In 1986 The World Health Organization met in Ottawa and released a Charter – The Ottawa Charter – that instigated the use of advocacy and empowerment for all, stating that all individuals should be able to make informed choices concerning their own care. Such decisions should apply whether the individuals were benefiting from health promotion or were choosing life-prolonging treatments in the terminal stages of an illness (Russell and Sander, 1998). Consequently the American Government produced the Patient Self-Determination Act 1990, which required that all medical staff and health care agencies provide adequate education and information concerning the patient's rights to formulate advanced directives (Wernow, 1994; Goetschius, 1997; Landry *et al.*, 1997).

No such document exists in British Law, although patients who can prove that they are 'competent' and fully informed have the 'right to refuse treatment' (Thompson, 1994; Lowe, 1997; Stauch, 1998). However, the present policy in all Accident and Emergency (A&E) departments throughout the country is to provide life-saving treatment for all attendees. Disclaimers, suicide notes and living wills are not accepted, and patients may have difficulty proving that they are competent to make a decision of that nature at that particular time (Toulson, 1996).

Advance directives

Advance directives (ADs) are documents in which individuals can lay out their personal wishes concerning their treatment should they be unable to make fully informed choices some time in the future. These include such methods as a living will, a living will card, and appointing a proxy.

A *living will* (see Appendix) requests and directs carers, usually health professionals, by consenting to or refusing treatment (Drain, 1993). The format is usually constructed to enable the individual to refuse specific treatments or medications (Berghmans, 1998). The Patients' Association (1996) suggests that one of two statements be used; a general statement made when the patient is in good health predicting for future mental or physical incapacity, and a specific statement. The latter statement should be completed only after a serious diagnosis has been made, and may include specific treatment options or indicate which treatments should be withheld. Each of these statements becomes operable when a patient is terminally ill (Perrin, 1997). The living will should always include the prefix 'I', as in me, and be signed by one or two witnesses who are capable of assessing the mental and emotional competence of the patient, although they need not be medically trained. Each AD should include a clause that allows the patient to withdraw the document at any time; this can be done either verbally or in writing (CARE, 1993; Patients' Association, 1996; Campbell, 1999). The instigator of the AD, the patient, should review the statement at least every 5 years, taking into account advances in medical technology and any changing circumstances and wishes.

The patient should keep the original document safely and inform relatives or friends of its whereabouts. Copies should be lodged with other relevant parties, such as the patient's general practitioner and the proxy, who is usually a relative or close friend. If hospital treatment is being provided, a copy of the AD should be included in the patient's medical records (Landry *et al.*, 1997). All health professionals who care for the patient should be aware of the existence and content of the AD (Perrin, 1997).

A *living will card* can be carried in the same way as an organ donor card, and should state clearly that the holder has a living will. It may also state that the holder does not want to be kept alive by artificial means (Davies, 1993). A contact number of a person who knows where to find the actual document should also be included on the card.

A *proxy* should be appointed by the patient while he or she is fully competent, and given power of attorney (Drain, 1993). The nominee, usually a close relative or friend, must have a good understanding of the patient's wishes, and have the patient's interests at heart (CARE, 1993; Patients' Association, 1996). This proxy is then able to support the patient's wishes whilst he or she is still able to make decisions, or enter into discussions concerning the patient's treatment options with health professionals if that individual becomes unconscious or incapacitated.

The living will (see Appendix), which may be completed years before illness or disability strikes, is probably the most controversial of the ADs. Rapid advances in medical technology create both advantages and disadvantages for those who have completed such a document (Wernow, 1994). Modern health care is at the mercy of technology as innovative treatments provide a wider range of choices for the consumer, and enable patients to survive with their disease or condition long after they would have died without medical intervention (Matzo, 1997; Berghmans, 1998). The general public believes that these interventions will prolong an individual's life span for an indefinite period, but believe that the quality of life may not always be improved and may, in many cases, be reduced (Russell and Sander, 1998; Eisemann and Richter, 1999). Perceptions of this nature have created a fear of being over-treated and left in an intolerable condition from which there is no chance of recovery (Patients' Association, 1996). The documentation of certain treatments that the patient desires to be withheld under specific circumstances provides the individual with some measure of control over and against technology (Fiesta, 1997).

Although the patient is able to make any preferences known in several ways, it must be made clear by all advisors that in British Law no such document is legally binding. However, the British Medical Association (1995) suggests that if the patient or other persons make a current legitimate document available to medical staff, the patient's wishes should be treated with respect. An AD will be considered invalid if it includes an unlawful request such as euthanasia. Specific treatments that have been documented can only be carried out if the physician feels they are in the patient's best interest (Calman, 1997).

Practice issues

This section considers the practical issues surrounding advance directives in practice. Client consent, empowerment and autonomy are explored, as is the effect of such a document on professional practice, with particular reference to the role of the advanced nurse practitioner (ANP).

The validity of the living will is centred on the patient's capacity to consent to or refuse treatment. If an AD has been signed in advance, the patient's competency may not be under threat. However, for those patients who are instigating a living will near the end of life, competency may well be challenged. In these circumstances the judgement of the health professional should be based on 'current practice and legal requirements' (British Medical Association, 1995, p. 26). Until recently, such decisions would be entirely in the hands of the attending doctor or consultant. As the role of the nurse expands in the form of the ANP current practices will change, and autonomous decisions are more likely to be made by the attending health professional, whether nurse or doctor.

The patient's competency may vary depending on drug regimens or levels of consciousness, and if these conditions are borne in mind it should be possible to discuss the patient's wishes when they are most lucid. The ANP is in an ideal position to judge whether the patient is able to understand and remember information. Nurses in regular and constant attendance are often able to communicate well with the patient and their relatives as they build up a relationship over a period of time. The ANP, with the support of nursing colleagues, will be able to provide full and understandable explanations at times when the patient is alert. It is important that the patient is given a full explanation and is able to understand and remember the information given about treatment choices, particularly in a situation where refusal or acceptance of treatment could precipitate death (British Medical Association, 1992; Greipp, 1992). Should a patient or relative later be able to prove that inadequate information was provided, the health professional could be exposed to a charge of negligence or battery.

Health professionals and carers may have a paternalistic attitude towards any decision made by the patient, concluding that if the patient agrees with the advice given then he or she is lucid, but when doubtful of options or refusing treatment the patient is 'incompetent'. Fisher *et al.* (1993) conclude that whether the patient's choice seems to be rational, irrational or have no reason, it should still be upheld. Many patients wish to discuss options with relatives, friends or their carers, particularly if any uncertainty exists; however, any undue influence from these sources may vitiate the consent (Richards, 1998; Stauch, 1998). Relatives may want to know more about the choices available to the patient. Nurses are always in attendance, and relatives will ask questions without wanting to bother the doctor. Facts and alternatives can be given by the ANP, who has a professional responsibility to keep the patient informed and act as an advocate. Sufficient time should be given to allow the patient to consider all options and thus make an informed choice, un-coerced by those present. If it is established that the patient is unable to give consent due to lack of consciousness or understanding, then a previously produced AD should take effect.

The proxy, relatives and health professionals should know the wishes and feelings (both past and present) of the patient, and take into account the factors that the patient would consider if able to do so (Hoyte, 1997a). British government reforms unveiled in October 1999 enable those appointed as proxy to have 'continuing power of attorney'. This allows the proxy decision-maker to take health care decisions for the patient, including consenting to the withdrawal of life-prolonging treatment (Dyer, 1999). The British Medical Association (1999) has published guidelines for doctors concerning life-prolonging treatment, and the withdrawing or withholding of treatment that has the potential to postpone the patient's death. These guidelines include advice on such controversial areas as artificial nutrition and hydration. However, they recommend that wherever possible an independent medical opinion should be sought or discussion with the friends or relatives should take place. Aarons and Beeching (1991) suggest that decisions concerning such important issues as resuscitation or further treatment should never be made independently. Each participant in the patient's care should be allowed to make a contribution in the decision-making process, thus providing a range of perspectives, which should result in a conclusion mirroring the patient's wishes. It is the ANP's responsibility as advocate to ensure that the wishes of the patient are fully considered and understood, and if possible implemented.

Caplan and Hansen-Flaschen (1997, p. 1532) state:

> . . . *any decision to violate a patient's wishes could be condemned as intolerable paternalism at best, manipulation, coercion or at worst assault.*

Consequently, any person who intentionally touches another person against his or her will, even if no harm is sustained, is trespassing and can therefore be sued for battery (McKee, 1999). If a living will has been produced, then any attempt to give treatment that has been specifically refused or to give treatment without the consent of the patient could well amount to a charge of battery, provided the mental competence and the level of knowledge of the individual were not in dispute at the time the AD was completed (Gilberthorpe, 1996; Hoyte, 1997b).

The general purpose of an AD is to allow patients to control the way in which they die. *The Patients' Charter* (DoH, 1992) publicized participation in patient care, emphasizing empowerment and autonomy in personal decision-making in relation to health care. The government's more recent white paper, *The New NHS: Modern, Dependable* (DoH,

1997), encourages the Health Service to become more sensitive and responsive to the needs and wishes of all patients and their relatives. Currently, the controversy surrounding the documentation and implementation of ADs seems to be in direct conflict with government policy.

British society actively encourages its citizens to make choices about every aspect of their lives except the way in which they die. Shaw (1997) questions the morals of a society that will take an individual's independence away at such an important time. Flanagan and Holmes (1999) suggest that many patients document their wishes because they are frightened of becoming dependent upon relatives or the state, and not because they are frightened to die. However, Caplan and Hansen-Flashen (1997) believe that patients' ability to control the nature and extent of their care has become an inviolable moral value. Stauch agrees, stating that 'every human being of sound mind and adult years has a right to determine what shall be done with his own body' (Stauch, 1998, p. 84). Nevertheless, whilst patients may be encouraged to determine the extent of their own treatment, this empowerment and autonomy should not give the individual the right to put other patients or carers at risk (Kjervik and Badzek, 1998).

Health workers have welcomed the ability for patients to become empowered and autonomous (Savalescu *et al.*, 1998). Indeed, the core concept within health care, and the central aim of nursing, is to allow patients to become autonomous and take responsibility for their own actions (Malin and Teasdale 1991; Singleton and McLaren, 1995; Morgan, 1996). However, many health professionals feel they are not adequately fulfilling their role as carers unless they 'take control'. This attitude results in an inability to allow the patient independence in even the most mundane tasks, and perpetuates the model of Parsons' (1951) 'sick role'. However, Seedhouse (1988) questions the ethics of allowing patients to decide on their own treatments, believing that physical and emotional stresses will prevent them from making appropriate decisions.

Kendrick states that many 'health professionals treat patients in a way which is analogous to the way parents treat a child' (Kendrick, 1994, p. 827), believing them to be unable to make informed decisions concerning their own care. This paternalistic view is shared by a number of health professionals who believe that the most appropriate decision is the one that they themselves would choose. Fisher *et al.* (1993) suggest these personal attitudes reflect those of society as a whole, which shows the desire to see life preserved. However, patients' wishes may be different to those of their health carers, as they will act upon their own conscience and personal views formulated from their earliest experiences and affected by present circumstances. Such views will have been formulated and influenced by societal differences, upbringing, personality, and spiritual and professional backgrounds (Mackie, 1977; Greipp, 1992; Penn, 1992). It is imperative that the professionals providing care should be aware of such differences, and try to understand a patient's point of view. This will give them some insight into the reasons for the acceptance or denial of treatment (Burnard and Chapman, 1988; Fisher *et al.*, 1993; Singleton and McLaren, 1995).

The United Kingdom Central Council states that nurses have a professional commitment to 'recognise and respect a patient's involvement in the planning and delivery of care' (UKCC, 1992), although Wright (1995) believes that many nurses are loath to surrender their control over patients. However, not withstanding this, nurses are ideally placed to understand the ideals and needs of patients. Holistic care provided by nurses incorporates all aspects of the individual; the mind, the body and the spirit. Each of these areas needs to be balanced, and the close, almost constant, contact between the nurse and each individual patient enables a unique relationship to be formed (Ellis, 1999). The experienced nurse uses each interaction to establish and maintain a good relationship, which supports, sustains and strengthens patients. Boykin and Schoenhoffer (1993) describe this interaction as 'interconnectedness' – a closeness that enables the nurse to listen and understand the wishes of the patient.

Those who have been diagnosed as having a terminal illness and those who are dying often feel vulnerable and unable to express or articulate their needs or wishes except to those close to them. However, they want to know that they will receive good nursing care and effective pain relief until the very end of life. The nurse has a special responsibility to maintain the dignity and respect of these patients and ensure that they do not suffer any unnecessary medical interventions (Riley, 1997; Wilks, 1999). The NHS declares that it is built around the needs of patients, not those of institutions, so it is able to provide a service that is sensitive and responsive to patients' needs (DoH, 1997). This admirable attitude needs to be acknowledged in many areas of the service, as the creation of dependency, paternalism and coercion, however subtle, is still rife (Gough, 1998). ANPs who act as advocates need to be aware of the environmental, economic and political forces that affect the treatment of their patients. These forces need to be reconciled with the needs of patients, consequently allowing communication to be a two-way process from the government to the consumer and *vice versa* (Hampton, 1993; Rafael, 1996; Kazanowski, 1997). In addition, ANPs must constantly be aware of any changes in legal guidelines. This current knowledge protects both the patient and the nurse from any deviation of patient care and a possible suit of malpractice.

Advocates should have a heightened awareness of their own attitudes and those of participating carers, as patients who have become dependent can easily be affected by the moral judgements and values of others (Jones, 1993). Projected values would not be true advocacy, but an equivocal act. Consequently nurses must be aware that they have a moral responsibility for their actions once they have accepted this role (Husted and Husted, 1991; Downie and Calman, 1994). Patient advocacy is not an intrinsic element of nursing, but any nurse who provides a holistic approach to patient care should be able to encourage and support patients in increasing their own well-being and exercising their freedom of self-determination (Gaylord and Grace, 1995). ANPs act as advocates not only for their patients but also for their colleagues, guiding and supporting them as they encounter attitudes and decisions that they feel unable to control.

Case studies

The following case studies highlight incidents in which knowledge of ADs is particularly relevant to the role of the ANP. All names have been changed to protect the identity of the patients.

Elizabeth

Elizabeth, an elderly Polish lady, has been a member of a health care practice for many years. During this time her health has steadily deteriorated so that now she is classed as disabled from her rheumatoid arthritis and chronic obstructive airways disease. She lives in sheltered accommodation with her small poodle, is fiercely independent and has a 'heart of gold'.

One morning she telephoned the surgery to request a visit as she had 'a little difficulty with my breath'. One of my extended dutie ⸻ ʲⁱⁿ the practice as an advanced nurse practitioner is to share the vi general practitioner – often an interesting and rewardin increases my understanding of my patients.

Elizabeth met me at her door; her chest was rattling, but normally if she called for a visit she would be so breathless that she couldn't move or talk. I noticed that Suki, her dog, was not threatening to trip her up, and asked her where she was. Elizabeth burst into tears, saying:

> *Suki too ill, you know. I can't look after her. She better dead. Me too. All my family going home to wedding. I too old, too tired to travel. If I dead I be scattered in beautiful place, be with my family. How can I get, you know, the injection?*

Sitting Elizabeth down I explained that euthanasia was illegal in this country, and that if you feel poorly everything else seems worse. If she felt better, she might change her mind about dying. I asked her if she was frightened of her forthcoming operation:

> *I not frightened of dying! I frightened of being kept alive on those breathing machines. Can't do anything . . . just like vegetable.*

We talked of the possibility of her being 'kept alive', of her family and friends, and the plans she had for the disposal of her remains when she died. Elizabeth seemed very adamant about the care she wanted both before and after her death. I asked if she had ever heard of an advance directive or a living will. I explained about the documents, and about how people were completing them because they had the same worries that she had expressed. I promised to let her have the address if she could contact me in the surgery. This would give her time to think about our conversation. Elizabeth recovered from her operation, and has since contacted me for more information about living wills. Should she complete the document it could, if she wishes, be stored in her notes at the surgery.

I feel privileged that Elizabeth felt able to talk to me in such an open manner, and hope that I will be able to continue to support her.

Malcolm and Edna

Malcolm and Edna are an articulate married couple in their late sixties who are still very much in love. They attended the surgery for blood pressure checks – Edna for her routine 6-monthly check, and Malcolm every fortnight as his previously well controlled hypertension had become labile. Although Malcolm had taken antihypertensives for some years, the onset of ischaemic heart disease had dramatically altered his previously active lifestyle. During previous appointments, Edna, Malcolm and I had explored their obvious anxiety and frustration about the disease and discussed ways in which they could chang activities to accommodate the restriction in Malcolm's ex tolerance and manage any symptoms he experienced.

Both Edna and Malcolm had completed living wills, and copies of documents had been inserted into their Lloyd George notes several years ago. I now felt they were ready to review the contents of the document, taking into account their change of circumstances. All advance directives should be reviewed regularly; a 5-year interval is suggested by the BMA, or less if there is a change in the patient's health status.

I approached the subject by reminding them that each of their notes contained such a document, and asked them if they could remember the date they had completed them. Such an approach enabled me to extract the documents and show them to Edna and Malcolm without it seeming to be a big issue. The living wills had been completed 3 years before. I was able to ask the couple how they felt, particularly now Malcolm had a heart problem which he had been told may mean major surgery – perhaps they would like to reconsider their position?

The couple had obviously considered the possibility of Malcolm's death, but remained adamant that the documents should remain as they were, both in substance and in the notes. I explained that the surgery should not be the only place to know about the existence of the living wills, and advised them to talk to the consultant who was looking after Malcolm's health, as he should also have a copy of the document. This they agreed to do.

Although I knew Malcolm and Edna well, I felt uneasy talking about the possibility of Malcolm's death whilst he was in such a vulnerable position. I believe this is due to the training all health professionals receive, which is to save life or extend its length until the very end. In contrast to this attitude, my position requires me to be an advocate for patients. Ensuring they have the opportunity to decide upon their future care enables this couple to remain in control and make decisions about their quality of life knowing each other's wishes.

Summary

Dying is often considered in a negative light; however, it should be a time when patients and their relatives are able to express their emotions of frustration, fear, anger and love without being judged. If patients are supported when they are developing their own personal coping strategies, they will have lower levels of stress, anxiety and depression. Consequently they will feel more able to make decisions and remain in control of their own treatment. Good, effective and honest communication between nurses, doctors, patients and their relatives is essential in order to maximize support, and this should occur whilst retaining the patient's dignity and independence. Patients who are able to discuss their treatment and their feelings openly without fear of being ignored or ridiculed are more likely to have their wishes understood and upheld, and documentary evidence in the form of an AD assists in this. However, if there is any question of the document being revoked, this should be considered seriously by all parties until the patient has made a final decision.

Many doctors or nurses may not feel comfortable with the idea of an AD being executed. Where these feelings are based on personal principles, health professionals should be able to arrange for other staff to provide care for the patient.

ANPs need to be aware of the legal and personal implications concerning ADs, and the effects that implementing these documents can have on staff and relatives. As an autonomous practitioner the ANP is in an ideal position to become an advocate not only for the patient and relatives, but also other members of staff who need support and information in this area.

Key points

- An AD is not a legal document in Great Britain.
- If an AD is produced, it should be treated with respect.
- Ignoring an AD may result in a charge of battery or assault.
- Specific treatments may be refused but not requested on the AD.
- An AD may be revoked at any time, either verbally or in writing.
- Any AD document should be witnessed by two independent people.
- All close relatives, friends and health care personnel should be aware of the presence of an AD.
- The original document should be retained by the instigator, and a copy should be kept with the medical records.
- The BMA recommends that an AD should be reviewed by the instigator every 5 years, or after a change in health circumstances.

References

Aarons, E. and Beeching, N. (1991). Survey of 'Do not resuscitate' orders in a district general hospital. *Br. Med. J.*, **303**, 1504–6.

Berghmans, R. (1998). Advance directives for non-therapeutic dementia research: some ethical and policy considerations. *J. Med. Ethics*, **24(1)**, 32–7.

Boykin, A. and Schoenhoffer, S. (1993). *Nursing as Caring: A Model for Transforming Practice*. National League for Nursing Press.

British Medical Association (1992). *Information on Advance Directives*. BMA.

British Medical Association (1995). *Advance Statements about Medical Treatment. Code of Practice*. BMA.

British Medical Association (1999). *Withholding and Withdrawing Life-prolonging Medical Treatment*. BMJ Publishing Group.

Burnard, P. and Chapman, C. M. (1988). *Professional and Ethical Issues in Nursing. The Code of Professional Conduct*. John Wiley & Sons.

Calman, K. (1997). On the state of the public health. *Health Trends*, **29(3)**, 67–79.

Campbell, N. (1999). A problem for the idea of voluntary euthanasia. *J. Med. Ethics*, **25(3)**, 242–4.

Caplan, A. and Hansen-Flaschen, J. (1997). Previous refusal of consent may not be relevant. *Br. Med. J.*, **315**, 1532.

CARE (1993) Living wills. The issues examined. *Ethics Medicine*, **9(1)**, 6–9.

Concise Oxford Dictionary (1964). 5th edn. Book Club Associates.

Concise Medical Dictionary (1980). Oxford University Press.

Davies, P. C. S. (1993). The right to die: who should choose? *Br. J. Nursing*, **2(13)**, 654.

Department of Health (1992). *The Patients' Charter*. DoH.

Department of Health (1997). *The New NHS: Modern, Dependable*. DoH.

Downie, R. S. and Calman, K. C. (1994). *Healthy Respect. Ethics in Health Care*, 2nd edn. Oxford Medical Publications.

Drain, G. (1993). Advance directives: partnership and practicalities. *Br. J. Gen. Pract*, **43(2)**, 169–71.

Dyer, C. (1999). Power of attorney change in England and Wales. *Br. Med. J.*, **319**, 211.

Eisemann, M. and Richter, J. (1999). Relationships between various attitudes towards self-determination in healthcare with special reference to an advance directive. *J. Med. Ethics*, **25(1)**, 37–41.

Ellis, S. (1999). The patient-centred care model: holistic/multiprofessional/reflective. *Br. J. Nursing*, **8(5)**, 296–301.

Farrar, A. (1992). How much do they want to know? Communicating with dying patients. *Prof. Nurse*, **7(10)**, 606–9.

Fiesta, J. (1997). Legal aspects of physician assisted suicide. *Nursing Management*, **28(5)**, 17–20.

Fisher, F., MacDonald, N., Western, M. R. *et al.* (1993). *Medical Ethics Today. Its Practice and Philosophy*. BMA.

Flanagan, J. and Holmes, S. (1999). Facing the issue of dependence: some implications from the literature for the hospice and hospice nurses. *J. Adv. Nursing*, **29(3)**, 592–9.

Freire, P. (1972). *Pedagogy of the Oppressed*. Penguin.

Gaylord, N. and Grace, P. (1995). Nursing advocacy: an ethic of practice. *Nursing Ethics*, **2(1)**, 11–18.

Gilberthorpe, J. (1996). *Consent to Treatment*. The Medical Defence Union.

Goetschius, S. (1997). Families and end-of-life care. How do we meet their needs? *J. Gerontol.*, **23(3)**, 43–9.

Gough, P. (1998). Commentary: Nurses should recognise patient's rights to autonomy. *Br. Med. J.*, **316**, 923.

Greipp, M. E. (1992). Greipp's model of ethical decision making. *J. Adv. Nursing*, **17(7)**, 734–8.

Hampton, S. (1993). Should euthanasia be legalised? *Br. J. Nursing*, **2(8)**, 429–31.

House of Lords (1994). *Report of The Select Committee on Medical Ethics*, Vol. 1. HMSO.

Hoyte, P. (1997a). Consent may not be needed to save life. *Br. Med. J.*, **315**, 1531–2.

Hoyte, P. (1997b). Writing medico-legal reports. *J. MDU*, **13(1)**, 18–20.

Husted, G. and Husted, J. (1991). *Ethical Decision Making in Nursing*. Mosby Year Book.

Jones, A. (1993). A first step in effective communication. Providing a supportive environment for counselling in hospital. *Prof. Nurse*, **8(8)**, 501–5.

Kazanowski, M. (1997). A commitment to palliative care. Could it impact assisted suicide? *J. Gerontol.*, **23(3)**, 36–42.

Kendrick, K. (1994). An advocate for whom – doctor or patient? How far can a nurse be a patient's advocate? *Prof. Nurse*, **9(12)**, 826–9.

Kjervik, D. and Badzek, L. (1998). Legal considerations at the end of life. *ANNA J.*, **25(6)**, 593–7.

Landry, F. J., Kroenke, K., Lucas, C. and Reeder, J. (1997). Increasing the use of advance directives in medical outpatients. *J. Internal Med.*, **12(5)**, 412–15.

Lascartos, J., Poulakou-Rebelakou, E. and Marketos, S. (1999). Abandonment of terminally ill patients in the Byzantine era. An ancient tradition? *J. Med. Ethics*, **25(3)**, 254–8.

Lowe, S. L. (1997). The right to refuse treatment is not a right to be killed. *J. Med. Ethics*, **23(2)**, 154–8.

Mackie, J. L. (1977). *Ethics: Inventing Right and Wrong*. Penguin.

Malin, N. and Teasdale, K. (1991). Caring versus empowerment: considerations for nursing practice. *J. Adv. Nursing*, **16(5)**, 657–62.

Matzo, M. (1997). Exploring the end-of-life issues. *J. Gerontol. Nursing*, **23(3)**, 7–8.

McKee, D. (1999). The legal framework for informed consent. *Prof. Nurse*, **14(10)**, 688–90.

Morgan, D. (1996) Respect for autonomy: is it always paramount? *Nursing Ethics*, **3(2)**, 118–25.

Parsons, T. (1951). Social structure and dynamic process: the case of modern medical practice. In: *The Social System* (T. Parsons, ed.), pp. 431–53. Routledge.

Patients' Association (1996). *Advance Statements about Future Medical*

Treatment. Patients' Association.

Penn, K. (1992). Passive euthanasia in palliative care. *Br. J. Nursing*, **1(9)**, 462–6.

Perrin, K. (1997). Giving voice to the wishes of elders for end-of-life care. *J. Gerontol. Nursing*, **23(3)**, 18–27.

Rafael, A. (1996). Power and caring: a dialectic in nursing. *Adv. Nursing Scientist*, **19(1)**, 3–17.

Richards, T. (1998). Partnership with patients. *Br. Med. J.*, **316**, 85–6.

Riley, B. (1997). Defining the core values of nursing, midwifery and health visiting. *Br. J. Community Health Nursing*, **2(10)**, 456.

Russell, P. and Sander, R. (1998). Palliative care: promoting the concept of a healthy death. *Br. J. Nursing*, **7(5)**, 256–61.

Savelescu, J., Marsden, R. and Hope, T. (1998). Respect for privacy and the case of Mr K. *Br. Med. J.*, **316**, 921–4.

Shaw, P. (1997). Dying with dignity. *Psychiatry Pract.*, **16(4)**, 16–17.

Singleton, J. and McLaren, S. (1995). *Ethical Foundations of Healthcare*. Mosby.

Seedhouse, D. (1988). *Ethics: The Heart of Healthcare*. John Wiley & Sons.

Stauch, M. (1998). Consent in medical law. *Br. J. Nursing*, **7(2)**, 84.

Thompson, M. (1994). *Teach Yourself Ethics*. Hodder and Stoughton.

Toulson, S. (1996). The right to die: the dilemma for A&E nurses. *Prof. Nurse*, **11(7)**, 435–6.

United Kingdom Central Council (1992). *The Code of Professional Conduct*. UKCC.

Wernow, J. (1994). The living will. *Ethics Med.*, **10(2)**, 27–35.

Wilks, M. (1999). Euthanasia: intent is the key issue, not outcome. *Br. J. Nursing*, **8(10)**, 634.

Wright, J. (1995). Can patients become empowered? *Prof. Nurse*, **10(9)**, 599.

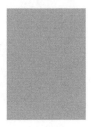

Appendix

The living will

THIS LIVING WILL is made on _____ Two thousand and one by
me _____ born on _____

I WISH these instructions to be acted upon if two registered practitioners are of the
opinion that I am no longer capable of making and communicating a treatment decision
AND that I am:

Unconscious and it is likely that I shall never regain consciousness, OR
Suffering from an incurable or irreversible condition that will result in my death within a
relatively short time, OR
Dependent on others for the rest of my life.

I REFUSE any medical or surgical treatment if;

Its burdens and risks outweigh its potential benefits, OR
It involves any research or experimentation that is likely to be of little or no therapeutic
value to me, OR
It will needlessly prolong my life or postpone the actual moment of my death.

I CONSENT to being fed orally and to treatment that may:

Safeguard my dignity
Make me more comfortable
Relieve pain and suffering,

even though such treatment might unintentionally precipitate my death.

SIGNED by me: _____

In the presence of
Witness signature: _____ Witness name: _____
Address: _____
Occupation: _____
Witness signature: _____ Witness name: _____
Address: _____
Occupation: _____

Index